The Most Powerful Constipation Natural Remedies Available

"Discover Constipation Cures Using Herbs, Juices, Fruits, Vegetables, and Food."

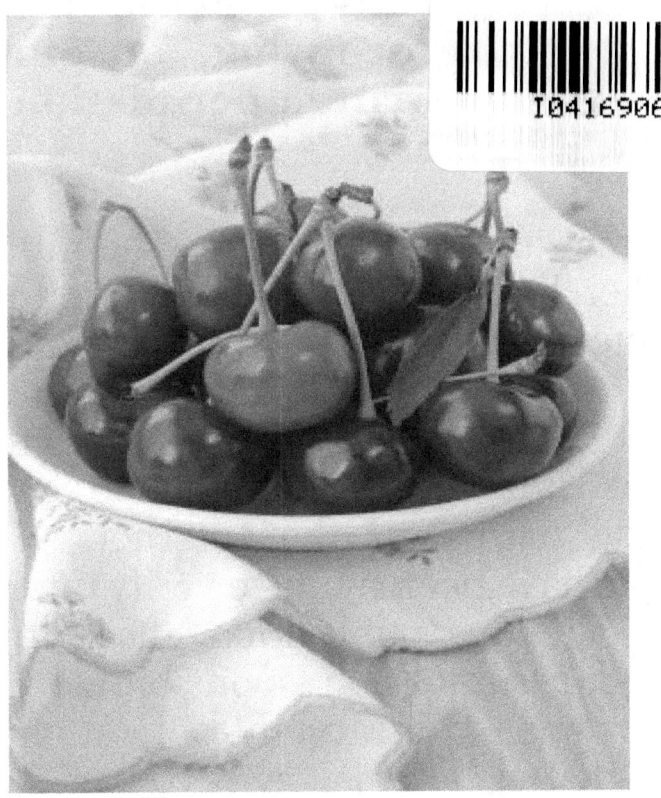

I0416906

By Christopher Teller, Natural Nutritionist

The Most Powerful Constipation Natural Remedies Available © 2014, by Christopher Teller

ISBN-13: 978-1503201163
ISBN-10: 1503201163

Disclaimer and Terms of Use: The Author and Publisher have strived to be as accurate and complete as possible in the creation of this book, notwithstanding the fact that he does not warrant or represent at any time that the contents within are accurate due to the rapidly changing nature of the Internet. While all attempts have been made to verify information provided in this publication, the Author and Publisher assumes no responsibility for errors, omissions, or contrary interpretation of the subject matter herein. Any perceived slights of specific persons, peoples, or organizations are unintentional. In practical advice books, like anything else in life, there are no guarantees of income made.

Your doctor or health provider should confirm any information given here. This information should not be taken as medical advice or treatment. This e-book is for information and educational purposes only. Consult with your doctor before using any of the remedies or information listed in the e-book.

Printed in the United States of America

Table of Contents

1: The Importance of Colon Health

I believe that to have good health we need to use mostly foods and supplements that are free of additives and food enhancers that are harmful to the body. We need to eat the right foods and watch how we prepare them so we can digest and absorb them without creating or leaving residues that get turned into toxic matter in our colon.

In this book, your will get some of the best constipation remedies that will help you overcome mild or severe constipation. For those of you who want to learn how to be free of constipation, this is the book for you. This information is based on my experience as a nutritionist and the work of many other nutritionist, naturopaths, and doctors.

The first question that a nutritionist or any other health practitioner should ask you on your first visit is, "how many bowel movements do you have each day or each week?"

If you visit a doctor now a day, your colon is the last area they discuss with you. And perhaps, this is an area they may never discuss with you at all.

In his article, The Bowel is an Ecosystem, in Healthy & Natural Journal, April 1997, Majid Ali, M.D. recounts,

"When I returned to the clinical practice of environmental and nutritional medicine after years of pathology work, I began carefully testing the assertions of nutritionists, naturopaths and clinical ecologist who claimed that various types of colitis a deterioration of your colon wall] could be reversed with optimal nutritional and ecologic approaches. To my great surprise, I found that such professionals, who are usually spurned by drug doctors, were right after all. My patients responded well to the unscientific therapies vehemently rejected by my colleagues in drug medicine."

Without good regular bowel movements and colon function, you will create various illnesses, colon discomforts, and diseases – including constipation.

By concentrating on eliminating constipation and preserving colon health, you have taken a major step in preventing many body conditions and illnesses that can shorten your life or make your senior years a miserable time.

If your colon is toxic, the blood will also be toxic. If your colon is toxic, these toxins will gradually reach all parts of the body through the blood and lymph liquid. The result is the body and various organs affected will become less efficient. Overtime this decreased efficiency will cause the body will become diseased.

By not eating clean food and without good colon health, you will be a victim of your own poisoning. It was estimated that of all the people who died of cancer – colon, lung, prostate, and breast - in 1999 sixteen percent were attributed to colon cancer.

This book will help you clear and eliminate constipation. It gives you information about your colon, so you can decide how to keep it clean and healthy.

It takes some work to do it. But you are going

to be eating, thinking, and living, so why not do it right and let go of the unhealthy habits. It is your choice. Now, take the right path. I am here to help you.

Do it one step at a time.

This book provides you with time-tested remedies that are all natural - foods, herbs, minerals, vitamins, and various nutrients.

Constipation is a warning your diet and lifestyle can be leading to some illness or disease in the future. It is a symptom that many people ignore or it is a symptom that many people try to eliminate by using unnatural dangerous laxatives.

Laxatives are probable the worst product you can use when you have constipation. They can become habit-forming if used too long and have some nasty side effects.

They have a tendency to create the problem you are trying relieve – constipation.

The remedies you choose to use will depend on specific herbs, foods, or nutrients you have, you can buy locally, you can buy on the Internet, nutrients you prefer, or you can afford.

Experimenting is part of how you find out what is best for you.

Keep in mind that all remedies listed here should be used only for a short time, two to four days and not longer than 2 weeks. They should only be used for the time needed to clear your constipation. Sometimes this might just be one or two times.

There are some herbal combinations you can use longer. These combinations can improve the health of your colon and get your bowels moving.

Look at the different remedies listed in the different chapters and use the one that feels right for you. Maybe it is the one where you have all the ingredients. Or, it could be the one you are familiar with the ingredients.

2: Fruit Juice Remedies That Eliminate Constipation

Fruit Juice Constipation Remedies

Ok let's get started. We are going to start listing the ways you can get relief from your constipation. For those who have been constipated for three to five days, you can use any of the methods listed.

Keep in mind that the simplest method can work, even with long term constipations. Each one of you is different and will react differently with specific remedies.

For Difficult Constipation Cases

For more difficult cases of constipation, sometimes more than one remedy might be necessary to relieve your constipation. From the list that follows you can use one remedy and if this does not work keep using this remedy but start using a second.

For Mild Constipation Cases

For cases of mild constipation, it may take a day or so to get your bowels moving again. For a more moderate case it may take 2-4 days. For a severe case it may take a week or so since your bowel wall may be weak and needs toning.

If you have diabetes or adrenal fatigue, limit your use of fruits and juices when you first wake up in the morning. However, exercise in the morning will help you tolerate drinking some juices in the morning

Organic Juices

Organic fresh made juices have cleansing and laxative action. These juices contain loads of mineral, bioflavonoids, vitamins, enzymes, antioxidants, and other nutrients. Citric fruits have citric acid and the more tart they are the more acid they have.

Fresh juice is a fast way to get all types of nutrients into the blood quickly. As juice nutrients get into your blood, they suck out toxics and build up tissues. In your colon they destroy bacteria, feed wall tissue, pull out toxins, and activate peristaltic action.

Even though juices provide helpful action throughout the body, it is best to limit their use and drink them in larger quantities only when trying to accomplish certain health benefits.

When juicing fruits and vegetables, the more fiber that is left with the juice the better results you will get with your constipation.

It is always best to use fresh juices, but as a last resort using packaged juices will be better than not drinking anything.

Apples and Apple Juice

Apples are good for eliminating constipation because they are high in pectin, a soluble fiber, have many minerals, and contain sorbitol - a natural sugar, which stimulates peristaltic action. Pectin helps to detoxify the intestines and promote regular bowel movements.

The fiber in apples adds weight and bulk to your fecal matter and helps draw water from your colon into the fecal matter keeping the stool from becoming hard and thus preventing constipation.

Apples are one of best fruits to eat because they are high in minerals, which provide alkaline electrolytes to your body. What this does is neutralize acids that are created during illness, anxiety, anger, exercising, breathing pollution, and improper eating. Body acid is a major reason we get deadly diseases as we age

Make eating apples or drinking fresh apple juice a daily habit. They are also effective in liver and gallbladder problems. .
Here's what to do.

Use crisp and hard apples such as granny smith, fuji, or gala for juicing.

Drink three glass of apple juice each day, morning, noon, and evening. In combination with drinking fresh apple juice, eat 3-4 apples each day to get fiber.

One-day apple and apple juice fast

You can also do a one-day apple and apple juice fast by,

Eat 3-4 apples during the day. Drink apples juice every two hours. Don't eat anything until the next morning. Then, start changing your eating habits as listed in the chapter 16.

If you do not want to do a one-day fast then eat your apples and drink fresh apple juice morning, noon, and night.

Apple cider vinegar

Take 1-2 tablespoons of apple cider vinegar with 8 oz. of water every day. And, add apple cider vinegar to your salad as part of your salad dressing. Just adding it to your salad will help to kill any bacteria or parasites that are in your vegetables. Apple cider vinegar will also kill any bacteria or parasite in your stomach that can cause you to have diarrhea.

Apple and Pear Juice

Prepare equal amounts of fresh apple and pear juice. Drink this combination when you first wake up and one hour before bedtime.

Juice the pears that are slightly hard. If the pear is ripe, it is best to blend it whole with apple juice to create a thick drink. Using the entire pear will give you additional fiber. Just remove the seeds, but do not peel the organic type.

Pears have minerals, vitamins, and chemicals that help to clean out your colon, kidney and to regenerate your blood cells.

Apple Juice and Prune Juice

If you have a juicer, you can make fresh apple juice and drink 3-4 glasses a day. You can also drink store-bought apple juice, but try to get fresh squeezed and not the type that has been flash pasteurized or pasteurized. If you can find fresh apple juice, then use flash pasteurized.

Buy your juice in glass containers if possible.

Plastic containers are processed using solvents that stay in the container walls and gradually outgas into the apple juice. This out gassing is more severe when plastic containers are stored in hot places.

To speed up the laxative effects of apple juice, take the following combination first thing in the morning before you have breakfast,

- Drink 2-3 cups of prune juice.
- After ½ hour, drink one cup of apple juice
- Then, 1-hour later drink another cup of apple juice.

I usually buy my prune juice in a bottle and fresh squeeze my apple juice.

Be prepared to head for the bathroom after you drink your prune juice and your first glass of apple juice. You may need to head to the bathroom soon after you drink prune juice, everyone is different. I have used this combination and have recommended it to my clients and have had good results.

Prune juice by itself is good for constipation. It is a safe, gentle and an effective laxative. Drink a cup in the morning and a cup in the evening. Prune juice contain the substance dihydrophenylisatin, which is responsible for the laxative action. Prunes are also high in iron and are a great supplement, if you are anemic or low on iron.

If you add prune juice to your diet, do not drink as much of it as you would when you have constipation. Drink ½ glass in the morning and perhaps ½ glass in the evening. Drink prune juice on occasion, but not regularly.

Apple Juice, Figs and Raisins

Here's another recipe using apple juice. Use it the first thing in the morning before breakfast.

In a blender, put in a cup of fresh apple juice. Add equal amounts of dry or fresh figs and raisins. Choose how many figs and raisins to use. You will need to experiment a little. Get a consistency that is not too thick. Add a little more apple juice if needed.

Oat Milk with Fig Juice or Prune Juice

Buy oat milk at the health food store. In the morning, warn 8 oz. of oat milk and add the following:

- 3 oz. of fig juice or prune juice
- two droppers full of licorice extract.

Or you can mix one glass of 50% fig juice and 50% prune juice. Drink this first thing in the morning.

Stewed Figs

Take 10 – 12 calimyma figs and stew them in two glasses of water (16 oz.) for 10 minutes. Let them sit in this water overnight.

In the morning remove the figs, warm and drink the juice. Eat the figs though out the day.

Or prepare a blended drink of,

- three or more figs, fresh or sun dried
- one banana
- 1 tablespoon of honey or molasses
- one cup of rice dream

Drink first thing in the morning and any time after lunch or dinner.

Mulberry Juice

Mulberry juice has many health benefits. It is good for digestive tract illnesses. It can stimulate digestion and assimilation of nutrients in the small intestine. It is useful for older people for reliving constipation.

Mulberry contains many minerals and vitamins.

Berries and Cherries

Boysenberry

Boysenberry juice has a gentle natural laxative action on your bowel. When your constipation is mild, this juice will help move things in your colon.

Blackberries

Mix ½ cup of distilled water and ½ cup of blackberries. Drink this first thing in the morning to promote peristaltic movement. Drink this often and it will make you regular. Blackberries are high in vitamin C.

Cherries

Cherries are high in antioxidants, fiber, potassium, and many other minerals, which are effective in neutralizing body acid. Cherries contain vitamin B-1, B-2, folic acid and niacin.

Cherries have laxative effects and can start

peristaltic action.

Eat fresh cherries throughout the day or drink three 8 oz. glasses of cherry juice during the day.

Buy cherry juice in glass container.
Elderberry Juice

These berries can be used to help reduce the symptoms of colds, flu, and also helps to relieve constipation, diarrhea, and hemorrhoids. Drink 1–2 glasses each day. Increase the quantity if necessary.

Citrus Juices

Citrus juices are an excellent way to stimulate your colon and other parts of the body. Since your colon is less active at night, drinking juices as soon as you awaken and get up can stimulate strong peristaltic action and promote a bowel movement.

Lemons

Lemons are filled with minerals, especially potassium, Vitamin C, and bioflavonoids. They have a cleansing action for the entire body.

Fresh lemon juice is the king of fruit juices. It contains citric acid, which acts in the body in a way no other juice does. First it acts on the liver to build up its enzymes so it can detoxify toxins in the blood. Then it combines with calcium to form soluble chemical substances. This makes it effective in removing kidney and pancreatic stones, plaque buildup along artery walls, and other calcium deposits that occur in the body.

When the liver, gallbladder, and pancreas are not working right, food digestion is affected. This in turn will create constipation.

Use lemons moderately since they break up oils during digestion and in our body making oils less available to our cells and joints.

If you have lemon allergies or ulcers then you should avoid lemon juice. If you have arthritis lemons are not a good choice.

Here's what to do:

Squeeze one lemon into a glass of warm distilled water. Drink it first thing when you wake up. Don't drink anything else for at least 1/2 hour.

You can use a citrus press to juice the lemon or just squeeze it to get the juice out.

Grapefruit Juice

Instead of drinking lemon juice, drink a glass of fresh squeezed grapefruit first thing in the morning. Again wait at least 1/2 hour before you eat anything.

If you are taking any anticonvulsant drugs, birth control pills, estrogen, protease inhibitors and even other types of drugs avoid drinking grapefruit juice. It slows the breakdown of certain drugs allowing them to increase in the blood to dangerous levels.

Grape fruit and Orange Juice

One drink I like in the morning is a combination of grape fruit and orange juice. Just prepare a half and half drink of these citrus fruits and drink it first thing in the morning.

Pineapple Juice

Drink a glass of pineapple juice first thing in the morning. Don't eat anything for at least half an hour. Then drink another glass at noon and just before you go to bed. Do this for the next three days.

Coconut and Carrot Juice

Mixing fresh coconut and carrot juice provides a tasty drink that has good laxative effects. Experiment with the amount of each juice you want to mix according to your taste. Drink this mixture for three days.

3: Powerful Fruit Remedies That Speed Up Your Stools

Fruits the Perfect Food

Fruits are made by nature and are a perfect food. They contain the right balance of nutrients with distilled water. You gain enormous benefits from eating fruits especially if you eat the outer skin. They are eaten without cooking. They are easy to digest and absorb and do not stress your colon.

Fruits contain fiber, which help to cleanse your colon and prevent constipation. Most fruits help provide the body with minerals that help the body reduce acid as it is created. And most important of all, fruits help cleanse the body of mucus slime that accumulates throughout the body.

Fruits do not leave any slime residue in the body when eaten except when they have pesticides and preservatives in their outer skin. They do not ferment or putrefy in your colon, as do processed foods, dairy products and meats.

Just Plain Fruits

Eat fruits throughout the day but especially in the evening. This will help to promote a bowel movement in the morning. These are the fruits you should eat.

- Apples
- Apricots
- Avocados
- Bananas
- **Blueberries**
- Boysenberries
- Cantaloupes
- Cherries
- Figs and dates
- Grapes
- Lemons
- Papayas
- Peaches
- Pears
- Persimmons
- Plums

- Prunes
- Raspberries
- Watermelon
- pineapples

Apples

Eat 3-4 apples a day to relieve constipation. It does not matter what type of apple you eat, but I like gala or fuji apples since they are small and crisp.

It is best to use fresh organic apples when eating apples as a snack since you will not know what pesticides were used in growing the apples. If apples are not organic, it is better to peel the apple before eating.

Using baked apples also helps to clear constipation.

Eat one baked apple at night, right before bedtime, and one just upon rising. Do this until you constipation is cleared.

In his book, John Heinerman, **Heinerman's Encyclopedia of Fruits, Vegetables and Herbs,** describes how to bake apples:

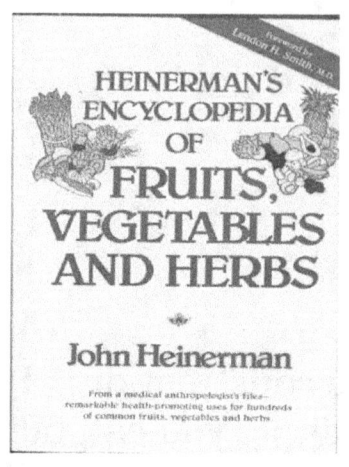

Cut apples in half and clear out the centers. Add chopped dates to the center. Pour some cranberry juice over the dates and apples. Then sprinkle cinnamon and nutmeg on the top. You can pour cranberry juice on some of the apples and see if you like the taste after they are cooked. Cook apples for 46-60 min at 375-400 C.

Dried Apples

Dried apple slices are also a good source of fiber. However, when the slices are dehydrated most nutrients are lost but fiber is retained. Sulfur dioxide is typically used to dry apple slices and this can cause allergic or asthmatic reactions in some people. I do not recommend using dried apple slices in place of fresh organic apples.

Just Apples and Mineral Water

Just after waking, eat two unpeeled apples, chew well, and then drink 8 oz. of water that has two drops of Alkalife. Or, you can use any other mineral additive or supplement you use.

This combination of apples and activated mineral water will stimulate your colon to become less sluggish and to move fecal matter out of the rectum.

I find Alkalife on e-Bay. This product cost $29.00 on the internet, but I have bought it for $17.00 on e-Bay.

Apricots

Apricots are one of most nutritious fruits since they are high in fiber, vitamin A, C, potassium, and have many other minerals. One apricot has around 1000 IU of vitamin A. This vitamin is mainly in the form of the precursor beta-carotene.

Apricots have a laxative effect and are usually available during the summer. Dried apricots are also good and are much higher in vitamin A and in minerals.

Use dried apricots that have not been dried with sulfur dioxide. Some people are allergic to sulfur dioxide and it is considered a pollutant that is found in our air. This chemical is a preservative that prevents apricots from turning brown.

If you have an ulcer, eating apricots with sulfur dioxide can increase your stomach acid and aggravate it.

Avocado with Apple Cider Vinegar and Lemon

Here's a recipe that will make you go to the bathroom in a couple of hours.

- Peel 1-2 avocados
- Add a little sea salt
- 3-4 tablespoons of apple cider vinegar (to taste)
- 1-2 tablespoons of lemon (to taste)
- Mix all together and spread on your favorite crackers
- Have a good time eating

Yes, avocados are high in fat but it contains the fat that is good for you, monounsaturated. In 4 oz., half of an avocado contains 500mg of potassium and folate.

Bananas

Bananas are rich in potassium. They assist in healing open wounds in the interior body membranes. They are helpful in stopping diarrhea and at the same time in promoting bowel movements.

Eat two bananas on an empty stomach followed by a glass of distilled water. After your constipation is cleared, eat only one banana each day.

Blueberries

Blue berries can act as a laxative for some people despite its use to stop diarrhea. These berries have chemicals, anthocyanosides, that can kill bacteria and viruses

Blueberries are also good for reducing inflammation. This makes them good for inflammations that occur all along the gastrointestinal tract.

Boysenberries

Boysenberry juice has a gentle natural laxative action on your bowel. When your constipation is not extra serious this juice will help move things in your colon.

Cantaloupe

Cantaloupe is one of best fruits you can eat. It contains many minerals and has Vitamin A and C. It is high in potassium. It has plenty of fiber and is useful for constipation.

Cherries

Cherries are high in potassium, fiber, and many other minerals, which are effective in neutralizing body acid. They contain vitamin B-1, B-2, folic acid and niacin.

Cherries have laxative effect and can start peristaltic action.

Eat fresh cherries throughout the day or drink 3 glasses, 8 oz., of cherry juice during the day. Buy cherry juice in glass container.

Dried cherries can also be used except the can be expensive.

Figs and Dates

Figs are high in fiber and can provide a gentle action on your colon when you have been constipated. This action can take about 24 hours before it takes place.

The use of figs and dates combined can have a stronger action on your colon.
Grapes

Grapes have a good laxative action. Eat 1-2 lbs. of grapes though out the day. Reduce the amount of food you eat during the day. Eat more vegetables and other fruits. Reduce the amount of processed foods you eat.

Grapes are high in vitamins and minerals. They have good fiber content and are especially high in manganese.
Since they are high in sugar, bugs are attracted to them. This causes farmers to spray them with pesticides. Try to find them at the farmers market as organic or not sprayed.

Papaya

Papaya is well known for its enzyme papain. Its minerals help reduce cell waste and eliminate stomach and colon mucus.

Persimmon

Eat 2-3 persimmons each day, if they are

available. They help to keep you regular.

Plums

Fresh plums are filled with minerals and have a mild laxative effect. They can relieve gas and have a cleansing effect on your intestines.

Prunes

Prunes are dried plums. Eat both for their natural laxative effect. Prunes are more effective than plums for constipation. Buy a bag of dried prunes and eat them throughout the day. Aside from this laxative effect, prunes are high in iron.

Raspberries

Raspberries are high in vitamins A and C. They are high in magnesium, calcium, and iron. They are helpful in clearing constipation.

4: Powerful Vegetable and Vegetable Juice Remedies

The benefits of Vegetables

Juices are absorbed quickly into your bloodstream. As a result, your cells are provided quickly with nutrients that feed them and that wash away waste. Juices give you the opportunity to get quick relief from various body conditions such as constipation. Juices move into your colon quickly to cleanse it and to activate peristaltic action.

Eating and drinking vegetables and their juices provide you with minerals and nutrients that build your blood, tissue, bones, and cells. It is minerals that build every part of your body. It is minerals that keep your body's pH at the required level. It is minerals that keep your body alkaline by neutralizing body acids.

It is minerals that build your colon wall tissues and cells so your colon can perform those activities that prevent constipation.

So, let's look at which vegetables and vegetable juices can help you end constipation.

Keep in mind that some natural recipes for clearing constipation require drinking vegetable juices that are bitter or have a strong taste. As you will find, some of the vegetable juices taste good and some don't. Remember you are dealing with a condition that needs clearing and that what you drink for this is not for pleasure.

As you drink some of these vegetable juices, you may find that you like certain ones and these can become your regular daily or weekly drink.

Rhubarb Mix

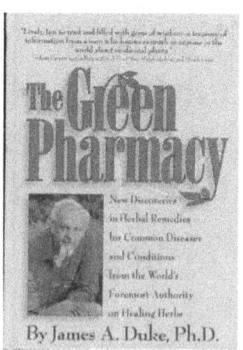

James A. Duke, PhD, in his book, The Green Pharmacy, gives the following constipation remedy using rhubarb.

"Rhubarb has strong laxative action so it is best to use it with other juices. Here's how you can use this herb. Blend together three stalks of rhubarb, without leaves, 1 cup of fresh apple juice, and one quart of peeled lemons and one tablespoon of honey or maple syrup. This tart drink will help you with your constipation.

Drink one glass three times a day."

A smaller quantity of this rhubarb drink would be, Blend three stalks of rhubarb, ¼ - ½ peeled lemon, a teaspoon of maple syrup, and ¾ cup of fresh organic apple juice. You may add more syrup if the taste is too harsh for you. Don't use rhubarb leaves since they contain toxic chemicals.

Use rhubarb only raw since it is high in oxalic acid. Use it sparingly and do not cook it. Cooking converts the organic oxalic acid into inorganic oxalic acid. The body does not easily absorb inorganic oxalic and it forms crystal deposits in the kidney and throughout the body.

If you have arthritis or gout, do not use rhubarb.

Carrot Juice

Carrot juices contain certain oils that work on the mucus membranes of the stomach and colon. This helps with digestion and starts your bowels functioning properly. Carrots are high in fiber and beta-carotene, an antioxidant, which the body converts to vitamin A. Carrots can make your stools softer and larger.

Why are larger stools better? Because larger stools dilute toxins, exposure less toxins to colon walls, and press against colon walls to promote peristaltic action.

Drink carrot juice twice daily, once in the morning and in the evening before bedtime.
You can drink more carrot juice if you like. Its action on the body produces enormous benefits since it contains a good number of vitamins and minerals – B, C, D, E, K, carotene, sodium, and potassium. These nutrients help to clean out your colon and speed up fecal matter movement.

As you increase the carrot juice you drink, chances are you will feel a little uncomfortable. This happens when carrot juice reaches your intestines and colon and begins stirring up the toxic layers and materials in that area. This feeling will pass and is nothing to worry about.

Carrot Juice, Carrots and Celery

An effective way to clear constipation is to combine vegetables that are high in fiber and that have laxative effects.

Celery is high in fiber, potassium, sodium, and many other minerals. It can reduces inflammation and protect against cancer. Celery has a chemical call polyacetylene, which reduces prostaglandins that cause inflammation.

Celery has a calming effect on the nervous system. If you have been using laxatives, which have overworked your colon nerves, celery will help to relax these nerves and give them a rest.

Adding carrot juice to celery juice provides an even better nutritional drink. This drink will help to restore nerve function in your colon and improve its health.

Here's what to do,

Eat carrots and celery during the day and for your salads; drink a glass of carrot juice in the morning and one in afternoon. By eating slightly steamed carrots you can increase the carotene available from the carrot by up to 4 times. However, by cooking carrots, you destroy the enzymes that will help you to digest them quickly and completely.

Boost your carrot juice by juicing with it a few stalks of celery which includes the leaves. The leaves have more nutrients than the stalk and are part of the nutritional value of the celery.

Tomato, Carrot, Celery Drink

Here's a drink you can take in the afternoon to activate a bowel movement.

With a juicer, juice some tomatoes, carrots, and celery. By experimenting you can discover the amount of each vegetable to use according to your taste. Mostly likely you will want equal amounts of tomatoes and carrots and you will want to add a few stalks of celery including the leaves.

Now, let's add a few more items to give your drink more pushing power. Squeeze in a small amount of garlic, onion, and radish. While juicing your carrots, juice a small bunch of spinach or parsley.

Drink 1 to 1 ½ cups in the morning.

Carrots, Cabbage and Raisins

Because carrots contain fiber, they help to form a good stool and promote peristaltic action. By combining carrots with cabbage and raisins, you can create an even more powerful food that will help in relieving constipation. Combine the following vegetables to form an evening salad:

Chopped carrots
Shredded cabbage (raw or slightly steamed)
Romaine lettuce
Cauliflower
Cucumbers
A handful raisins
Sprinkle a tablespoon of grounded flax seeds
Mix in 1 – 2 tablespoons of olive oil
Mix in 2 tablespoons of apple cider vinegar
One tablespoon of lecithin granules

Eat this salad once or twice a day for three days. After that you should continue to eat a vegetable salad for lunch or dinner.

Carrot and Spinach Juice

Combine 10 oz. of carrot and 6 oz. of spinach juice. Drink two pints daily. Both these vegetables have nutrients to help relieve your constipation.

Cucumber

Cucumbers are good for preventing constipation. But they can be used in the carrot-spinach juice or the apple-spinach juice. Cucumbers make these juices more powerful. Use only about ¼ - ½ of a cucumber when adding it to these juices. You can experiment with how much cucumber you want to add.

Cucumbers are a natural diuretic and help to dissolve kidney stones. Because they are high in potassium, they help to promote the flexibility of colon cells. This helps to keep your colon working, as it should.

Cabbage and Asparagus

Cabbage is high in fiber and contains a good amount of potassium, foliate, beta-carotene and many other nutrients – bioflavonoids, indoles, genistein, monoterpenes. It is these various chemicals that give it its potent ability to reduce or prevent colon cancer and heal various ulcers along the gastrointestinal tract.

Cabbage is anti-bacterial and helps to heal tissues in the stomach, intestines, and colon. Drinking cabbage juice produces intestinal gas. This gas occurs when cabbage juices combine with putrefied layers in the intestines and colon.

Use little or no salt on any preparation of cabbage. Salt destroys the nutritional value of cabbage.

There are many forms of cabbage you can use for your juices – green, red, savoy, bok choy.

Asparagus

Asparagus are also high in fiber. They also provide foliate and vitamins A and C. Refrigerate asparagus quickly if you are not going to use them and keep them for 3 days or less. Asparagus that have not been refrigerated lose their nutritional value quickly.

People with gout should not eat asparagus since they contain purines that can start a gout attack.

With a slight amount of water, steam, for 3-4 minutes, abbage and asparagus in a glass pot. Eat just before going to bed.

Beets

Beets are high in fiber, organic sodium, potassium, Vitamins A and C, iron and calcium. If you like beets, eat 2 raw beets in the morning and expect to have a bowel movement 10-12 hours later.

Cabbage and Beets

Blend 1/3 part beets and 2/3 part cabbage. Drink this mixture on an empty stomach. This is a strong tasting drink, but the cabbage contains a cleansing enzyme, lysozyme, which absorbs bacteria and toxins. This toxic material is eventually moved out in the fecal matter. Beets also promote bowel movements.

Cabbage and other juices

To make cabbage juice tastier, mix it with celery stalk and leave juice, tomato juice, and a citrus juice or pineapple juice. This juice can be used in the morning or evening.

Make a cabbage soup with ginger

Sauerkraut Juice

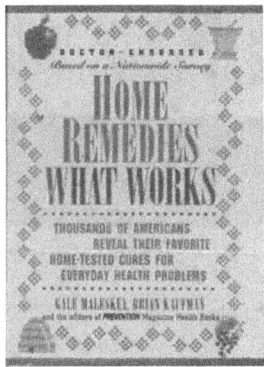

Sauerkraut juice has long been a remedy used by many people who have been constipated.

In their book, Home Remedies What Works, Gale Maleskey and Brain Kaufman, discuss sauerkraut juice.

"'I've used sauerkraut juice many times to relieve constipation of five or six days' duration, and it has always worked for me,' says Jacqueline, 49, a Floral Park, New York, housewife.

She picked up the re remedy from her father, who used to drink sauerkraut juice regularly. 'He lived to be 86 years old and never had any health problems,' she says.

She simply drains the juice - usually about ¾ cup – from a large can of sauerkraut, then drinks it. 'For me it works as well as milk of magnesia. I can count on results in about 1 to 1 ½ hours.' She's not alone. Several other people said sauerkraut juice is an effective laxative"

Sauerkraut juice should not be used regularly since it is high in salt. The salt helps to pull water into your colon, which helps to relieve constipation. In this process, electrolyte minerals are also flushed out.

Regular use of sauerkraut can deprive the body of vitally needed minerals and cause a health problem.

Sauerkraut and Tomato Juice

Perhaps a more tolerable drink using sauerkraut is to prepare it as follows:

Mix equal parts of sauerkraut and tomato juice. Add a touch of lemon and drink this twice a day, once in the morning and then in the evening.

Sweet potatoes

Sweet potatoes can help get you regular. Prepare sweet potatoes just before you go to bed. Boil or bake the sweet potatoes. Then eat them with some add milk, some salt, honey or sugar. This mixture for sure will get your bowels moving.

Corn

Cook corn for about 5-7 minutes. Don't overcook it. This will provide you with a great source of fiber. Eat more cooked vegetables until your constipation is cleared. But be sure to just cook them for a few minutes to soften them slightly. Cooking them too long makes the fiber too soft and less effective in your colon.

Greens

In a pan add some water with one or more teaspoons of olive oil. Turn the heat on and sauté some garlic. Now add small pieces of chopped broccoli. Cover and cook for around two minutes. Next add a bunch of spinach, chard, collard greens or kale, which ever greens you like. Cook for a few minutes. Add some water or oil as needed.

Serve with a pinch of apple cider vinegar, lemon juice, or balsamic vinegar. Add a bit more olive oil, or flax seed oil.

This provides an excellent source of fiber, chlorophyll, good oil, and minerals to help clear your constipation.

Another Green Remedy

In boiling distilled water, add mustard greens, collard, chard, and turnip leaves. Any three will do. Allow to cool slightly. Then eat the greens and drink the water. This will promote a bowel movement.

Endive Leaves

Endive lettuce has a bitter taste. However, its juice is good for clearing constipation. Use this juice in small quantities with other juice mixtures. Mix it with a carrot, spinach and apple mixture

Radish with Sesame oil

For constipation, mix 2 tablespoons of grated radish with one tablespoon of sesame oil. Take this daily to clear your constipation.

Parsnips

Parsnips contain more fiber than most other vegetables. This makes it ideal for helping clear your constipation. Use small ones since they are tenderer than large ones.

Parsnips are also high in potassium and contain chemicals that neutralize carcinogens in the small intestine and colon.

5: Fruit & Vegetable Remedies That Create Peristalsis Action

Apple Juice and Spinach Juice

Here's a recipe that I recently found in **Heinerman's Encyclopedia of Healing juices, 1994**. Heinerman says to, **mix equal parts of apple juice with spinach juice.**

I use one or two small apples and one bunch of spinach. Spinach does not have a strong taste for me so I only use one apple. But if it does for you, then use two apples or more to make this drink tasty.

Take two cups each day, one in the morning and one in the evening. Continue taking this mixture for about two weeks. After this time, evaluate how you feel and decide if you want to continue taking this mixture. If so, use this drink at a reduced interval – twice a week or once a week.

What I have experienced with this mixture is

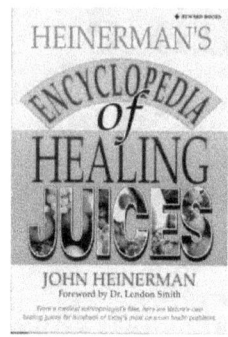

after 3-4 days of use, my bowel movement in the morning comes out in five seconds and that's it. Then I'm ready for my shower.

Here's what Heinerman says about this apple/spinach combination, "I've put many clients on two cups of this apple-spinach juice each day for up to a week and have had testimony after testimony come back to declaring how the most difficult cases of constipation, which no laxatives could begin to touch, had suddenly cleared up within a matter of days!"

In addition, Heinerman claims that this juice combination has a cleansing action on your bowel walls. It helps to remove some of the encrusted fecal matter that collects on your colon wall over the years.

Raw spinach juice is high in oxalic acid, which binds with calcium in the body when it is cooked. Even though you use it uncooked, in this recipe, I still recommend you take a calcium supplement with this apple/spinach combination.

I recommend 1:1 magnesium: calcium

combination of about 600-800 mg. For good intestinal absorption of these minerals, use Calcium Aspartate, Calcium Lysinate, Calcium Citrate or a combination of all three.

Notice that I recommend using a 1:1 ratio, which give equal amounts of magnesium and calcium. Most combinations you find in health food stores provide these minerals in a 1:2 combination. This combination gives twice as much calcium as magnesium. It is better to have equal amount of calcium and magnesium since magnesium is necessary for proper absorption of calcium.

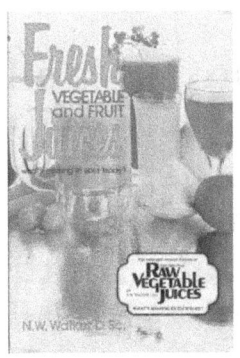

N.W Walker D.Sc., in his book, Fresh Vegetable and Fruit Juices, 1978, says, "Organic oxalic acid is one of the important elements needed to maintain the tone of, and to stimulate peristalsis...oxalic acid in our raw vegetables and their juices are organic, and as such are not only beneficial but essential for the physiological functions of the body.

The oxalic acid in cooked and processed foods,

however, is definitely dead, or inorganic, and as such is both pernicious and destructive.

When the Oxalic acid has become inorganic by cooking or processing the foods that contain it, then this acid forms an interlocking compound with the calcium even combining with the calcium in other foods eaten during the same meal, destroying the nourishing value of both. This results in such a serious deficiency of calcium that it has been known to cause decomposition of the bones.

This is the reason that I never eat cooked or canned spinach."

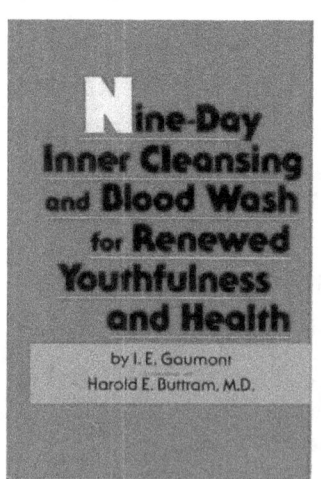

I.E. Gaumont and Harold E. Buttram, M.D also recommend spinach for constipation. In their book, Nine-Day Inner Cleansing and Blood Wash for Renewed Youthfulness and Health, they say,

"SPINACH is a protective food, particularly for the glands. A high source of vitamin A, and rich in chlorophyll, it is helpful in high blood pressure, functional heart trouble, anemia... It is indicated in medical circles that raw spinach juice taken in quantities amounting to about one pint daily has often corrected the most aggravated case of constipation in a short period of time."

Spinach is the riches plant source in folic acid and shortage in this vitamin can create constipation. It is also high in antioxidants, beta and alpha carotene, lutein and zeaxanthin as well as potassium, magnesium, vitamin K.

Celery, Spinach, grapefruit drink

Here's another juice drink you can make using spinach. Mix a combination of spinach, celery, and grapefruit juice. Drink this first thing in the morning.

Sauerkraut and Grapefruit Juice

This is a fast working remedy, if you have a blocked colon.

Drink 8 oz. of warm sauerkraut juice Follow this with 8 oz. of warm grapefruit juice

Be ready to head for the bathroom.

If this fails to rush you to the bathroom, try this combination again 45 minutes later.

You can also use just plain sauerkraut for constipation. Eat sauerkraut each day for 5 days each week.

6: Special Herbal Constipation Remedies Secrets

Herbal Remedies

Herbal laxatives help to promote bowel movements and relieve constipation. They remove food and toxic build up along your colon walls. When used in combinations, more than one herb, herbs provide nutrients and substances that help to feed and tone your colon walls and at the same time move fecal matter out through the rectum.

Strong Herbal Laxatives

Herbal laxatives can be weak, moderate, or strong. Strong laxatives are called cathartics or purgatives and are used when you have a severe case of constipation. The strong herbs are Aloe, Buckthorn, Cascara Sagrada and Senna.

They work by stimulating or irritating your

colon wall nerves, which promote a strong peristaltic movement.

Care must be taken when using strong laxatives since they have an irritating effect on your colon walls and some time can be painful and griping. As with drugstore laxatives, these strong herbs can create a lazy colon requiring you to use them over and over to have a bowel movement.

You will find some herbs mixed in with drugstore laxatives.

Weak and Moderate Herbal Laxatives

The best herbal laxatives to use are those that promote digestive juice secretions, which activate a bowel movement. Moderate herbal laxatives are herbs like licorice, Wahoo, Yellow Dock, Balmony, Barberry, Dandelion Root, flax seeds, and pysillium seeds.

Some herbal combinations are listed below that combine weak, moderate, and strong herbal laxatives. These combinations provide the benefits of both herbs and reduce the strong effects of the individual herbs.

Preparing Herbal Teas

When preparing a herbal tea, called an infusion, it is best to only use a glass, porcelain-lined or stainless steel pot with a cover. Boil distilled water, then, remove the pot from the stove. Do not use a microwave to heat your water. Microwaves change the electrical characteristics of water.

Place the herbs into hot water and stir. Cover the pot and let it sit for 5-30 minutes. The longer herbs sit in the water the stronger the tea becomes. After the tea cools a bit, strain it and it is ready to drink. If the tea is too bitter for you, you can add a touch of honey.

Use one teaspoon to one tablespoon of mixed herbs to 1 ¼ cup of distilled water.

If you are pregnant, do not use any of herbs listed in this chapter, since they are designed to promote contractions in your colon and surrounding areas.

Children's Herbal Dosage

When giving children herbal products use more care. Give a reduced amount based on the adult dosage.

Children's Age	Herbal Dose
10-14 years	½ adult dose
6-10 years	1/3 adult dose
2-6 years	¼ adult dose

Licorice Root

Licorice root has a mild laxative effect. It is good for ulcers and inhibits the growth of harmful viruses. It has high sugar content, so diabetics should use it with caution.

Licorice makes your body hold water. Do not use Licorice if you have high blood pressure, are pregnant, or use corticosteroid drugs. Licorice root may increase the side effects of these drugs.

If using digoxin, or diuretic drugs do not use licorice root since it pushes potassium out in the urine. DEGLYCRRHIZINATED, DGL, may be O.K. to use with this drug but check with your doctor to make sure.

Prepare 1 cup of tea using one tablespoon of

licorice root. Drink 3 times each day.

Anise seed tea

Anise seeds produce a tea that can improve your digestion, which helps to reduce constipation. Anise seed tea is also good for improving memory, brain activity, and overall body health.

Take two tablespoons of anise seeds and put them into a coffee grinder. Press the start button for 2-3 second just to break up the seed lightly.

Make a tea with these seed as follows:

Boil 1 ½ cup of distilled water in a glass pot. Pull the pot off the stove and put the seeds into the water and cover the pot. Let the seeds sit in water for 10-15 minutes to make a good strong tea.

Drink one cup of this tea first thing in the morning.

Alfalfa Tea

Alfalfa helps to relieve constipation. It is rich

in fiber, minerals, and chlorophyll. It is helpful in improving gastrointestinal function.

Warfarin and alfalfa interaction – Alfalfa is a high source of vitamin K, which helps blood to clot. This has the opposite of effect of the drug Warfarin, which helps to thin the blood to avoid clotting. If you are under a doctor's care and using Warfarin consult your doctor before using Alfalfa herb.

Alfalfa has many minerals so it is considered an alkalizing food. It contains C, E, K, and B vitamins making it one of the best herbs for building the body back to health.

Since alfalfa helps reduce infections, it is useful in infections that occur in your colon and throughout the body.

Prepare a cup of tea, using a tablespoon of alfalfa leaves. Let sit it for 10 –15 minutes. This tea has a strong grassy taste and you may want to add a bit of honey or lemon to reduce its strong taste.

Elderflower

Drink a tea of elderflower daily to relieve constipation

Chickweed

Drink 1 cup of chickweed every 3 hours. Do these until you have bowel movement.

Chinese Rhubarb

Chinese rhubarb, rhubarb, turkey rhubarb has been used for many decades to relieve constipation in China. It has a strong purgative action – it encourages strong laxative stimulation. It should be combined with other herbs, which reduces its purgative strength.

Pregnant women should not use Rhubarb.

Rhubarb, Ginger, licorice Infusion

For severe constipation, prepare an infusion of,

- 1 teaspoon of rhubarb powder
- ¼ teaspoon of ginger root
- ¼ teaspoon of licorice root

Drink 1/2 cup of this infusion and over a few days increase it to a cup.

Bentonite

Bentonite is clay from volcanic ash. It is used to cleanse your colon walls and can be used as a laxative. You will see it as an ingredient in some natural laxative formulas.

Butternut Root Bark

Butternut root bark is considered one of the safest laxatives. This following formula is a gentle but effective laxative herb combination.

- Butternut root bark
- Cascara sagrada bark
- Rhubarb root
- Ginger root
- Licorice root
- Irish moss
- Cayenne

This combination, with butternut, is listed in **a book called, The Scientific Validation of Herbal Medicine, 1986, by Daniel B. Mowrey, Ph.D where Mowrey say, "this**

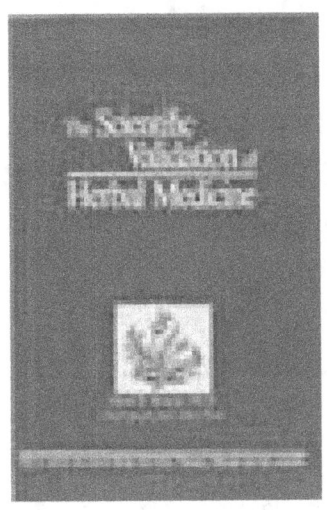

combination is due to the effectiveness of Butternut Root Bark – a mild and effective laxative – and Cascara Sagrada – one of the most effective herbal laxatives around and in addition helps to return the natural tone of your colon.

Ginger Root contains an oil called Ginerol which helps to bind the other herbs together and deliver them into your colon which they can assist in normalizing your colon."

Chamomile

Chamomile tea is often used as a relaxant and is useful in reducing tension, which can lead to a tight colon. It has a gentle laxative action and helps in digestion.

Drink one cup just before bed time.

Cayenne

Cayenne is effective in producing peristalsis in

your colon by aiding in digestion and stimulating elimination. It can be used regularly and when needed for constipation. Cayenne pepper is known to help thin the blood. So, it is good for improving the blood circulation.

Cayenne is available in capsules of different strengths, from 5,000 heat units (HU) to 100,000 and even higher. In addition, cayenne when used with other herbs helps to deliver these herbs more efficiently to where they are needed in the body.

Start with one capsule of 40,000 HU and always take it after you eat. You will feel a hot or slight burn feeling in the upper stomach and that's when you know it's working. The feeling I get is like when I get heartburn. This burning sensation will pass as your body gets use to you using cayenne.

Do not use cayenne seeds, as they can be toxic. If you are pregnant or breast-feeding do not take cayenne supplements. Use cayenne only as showed on containers and only as capsules.

Use the recommended dose shown on the

bottle of cayenne you use.

Cascara Sagrada

Cascara Sagrada comes from the bark of the buckthorn tree. It stimulates your colon to produce stronger contraction than normal. It can work on the most difficult cases of constipation.

It is one of the best herbs with a strong laxative effect. It will be found in many herbal combinations that are mixed for constipation. Cascara has Chrysophanic acid, which stimulates your colon wall to produce peristaltic action. Cascara also contains a chemical called emodin which controls the strong action of Chrysophonic acid thus producing a balanced laxative effect.

If you use cascara in a herbal mixture, do not use this mixture for more than thirty days. Then take a rest from it. Do not use Cascara in large amounts and for long periods since it can cause intestinal distress and become habit-forming.

Cascara Sagrada also stimulates secretions from the liver, gallbladder, pancreas, and stomach. These secretions give Cascara additional laxative effects.

Do not use Cascara Sagrada if you have irritable bowel syndrome, hemorrhoids, or ulcers. Use Cascara for a limited time. It can become habit-forming and, if used for an extended time, it can increase the risk of colon cancer. Its use also causes you to lose potassium with each bowel movement.

If you have liver problems do not use cascara sagrada full strength. Use it in combination with other herbs. Cascara is known to put a strain on the liver.

You can take cascara as a single herb. As a single herb, it can cause cramping and nausea. However, I recommend you used it with other herbs. In a herbal combination, the combination can detoxify your colon, tonify your colon walls, cleanse the blood and produce other synergistic actions.

In Michael Murray, N.D., book called The Pill Book Guide to Natural Medicines, he talks about the drug interaction of cascara sagrada,

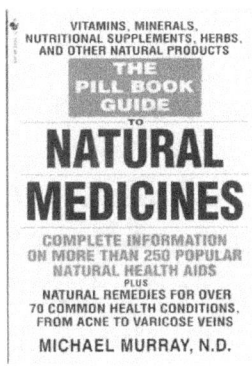

VITAMINS, MINERALS, NUTRITIONAL SUPPLEMENTS, HERBS, AND OTHER NATURAL PRODUCTS

THE PILL BOOK GUIDE

TO

NATURAL MEDICINES

COMPLETE INFORMATION ON MORE THAN 250 POPULAR NATURAL HEALTH AIDS

PLUS

NATURAL REMEDIES FOR OVER 70 COMMON HEALTH CONDITIONS, FROM ACNE TO VARICOSE VEINS

MICHAEL MURRAY, N.D.

"Cascara and other stimulant laxatives may decrease absorption of other drugs that pass through the gastrointestinal tract. If you are currently taking an oral medication, talk to your pharmacist or doctor before self-medicating with cascara.

Cascara may potentiate the action of digoxin and other heart medications due to potassium depletion. The use of cascara with thiazide diuretics and corticosteroids may further decrease potassium levels."

Recommend dose for the cascara, as a single herb, is 350 – 1000mg just before bedtime.

Use 1-4 cascara powder capsules a night, but do not use these capsules for more than 10 days. Start with 1 capsule a night and increase the amount each day until you get results you want.

For a laxative tea, use one teaspoon of cascara bark in 3 cups of boiling water for 30 minutes. Drink 1-2 cups of tea just before bedtime after it has cooled to room temperature.

Dandelion

Dandelion has a laxative action and helps to resolve mild cases of constipation and stomach aches. It also has a blood cleansing effect and helps to detoxify the liver kidney, gallbladder, pancreas and the stomach.

Use 1 cup of Dandelion tea, with a touch of honey, 3 times each day.

If you have problems with your gallbladder in any form, it is best not to use dandelion. It has a detoxifying effect on the gallbladder encouraging bile flow.

Recommend dose is 200-250mg each day.

Senna

Only use senna for a short time, 1- 1½ week. It is not healthy to use it for a long time since its action moves fecal matter through your colon quickly. This quick action prevents absorption of nutrients by your colon depriving you of necessary minerals and vitamins.

Use senna only in amounts that produce the required bowel movement and stool softness to relieve your constipation. Start with small amounts and increase your amount slowly.

Senna is sold Over-the-Counter under the name Correctol®, ExLax®, Senokot®, and Smooth Move. Senokot also contain docusate sodium - a stool softener - an added benefit when hard, dry stools may cause discomfort.

Seena Tea

You can also prepare a seena tea as follows:

Buy some seena tea at a health food. Place a tea bag into 1 ½ cups of distilled water and steep. Then, add the peel of a whole red potato. Also, add a couple slices of potato meat. Add to this, a teaspoon of wheat or oat bran and flax seed.

Simmer this combination, strain it and drink the liquid. This will help some of the more difficult cases of constipation. Remember the longer you simmer this combination the stronger the tea will be. Start with a 5-10 minutes and then work up to 15-20 minutes but you need to experiment with the time.

When you drink seena tea, drink only 2-3 oz. at a time and drink it only after it has cooled down. It has less of a cramping action when you drink it cool.

Seena Tea with Mint

Here is another seena tea you can prepare.

1 teaspoon of seena tea leaves
½ teaspoon of peppermint leaves.

Boil 8 oz. of distilled water, turn the heat off, stir in the herbs. Turn the heat off and cover the glass container. Let tea simmer for 3-10 minutes.

Add honey to improve taste and some powered vitamin C if you have it.

Look for formulas that have a small amount, 1/10 of a part, of fennel, anise, or ginger to reduce any cramping that might occur with seena.

Do not drink seena tea or capsule if you have any type of colon disease, stomach pain, diarrhea, or are pregnant.

Senna Pods are milder than the leaves since the do not contain resin. It is the resin in the senna leaves that causes griping in your colon.

If available, use around 8 pods. Heat some distilled water. Place the pods into the water for 5-10 minutes. Strain the tea and add 3-4 dried prunes or chopped prunes. Let cool and eat the prunes during the day or drink and eat a few prunes just before you go to bed. Drink only a couple ounces of the senna liquid at one time. If cramping or griping occurs, reduce the amount of tea you drink.

Psyllium

If you have asthma, do not take or use psyllium. Some people with asthma have had allergic reactions to psyllium and the powder from psyllium can cause an asthma attack.

Some you may be allergic to psyllium. If you are, you may become constipated or develop dark areas under your eyes.

In your colon, psyllium activates peristaltic action and helps to clean your colon of any stagnation that has occurred there. By adding moisture to dry hard fecal matter, psyllium helps to move fecal matter through your colon. As psyllium seeds bulk up in your colon, they push against your colon walls stimulating peristaltic action. The soluble fiber in psyllium provides food for good bacteria, which helps them to multiple.

Here's how to use it:

For mild constipation, take 1 **tea**spoon in a glass of juice or warm water three times a day.

Work up to taking one teaspoon of psyllium by starting with ¼ teaspoon in a glass of water or juice, the next day ½ teaspoon and so on until you are taking one teaspoon. Do the same when considering taking up to two teaspoons of psyllium.

Start by taking one teaspoon just before going to bed. After drinking your glass of psyllium seeds, follow this up each time with another 8 oz. of clear distilled water.

For moderate constipation, take two teaspoons

in a glass of juice or warm water daily. Start by taking two teaspoons at breakfast time.

It can take up to three days to get relief and that depends on the dose you take.

Use psyllium seeds with care. Some cases have been found where psyllium seed parts have lodged in your colon wall, causing an irritation. When using excessive psyllium seeds, it is possible that it can deposit on your colon wall if you already deposited toxic waste there. This adds to the encrustation along your colon wall.

Continue to drink water during the day, up to 8 glasses a day, when using psyllium seeds. This helps push the seeds through your colon and not deposit along your colon walls. Remember the seeds bulk up and absorb water and you don't want them to cause constipation by bulking up and getting stuck in your colon.

Use psyllium seeds only long enough to relieve your constipation. Excessive use of psyllium can cause allergic reactions and can cause constipation, if used incorrectly.

Agar-Agar and Psyllium seeds

Agar and Psyllium seeds are mostly soluble fiber, which absorb a lot of water and bring it into your colon. This creates bulk in your colon, which puts pressure on your colon walls leading to peristaltic movement.

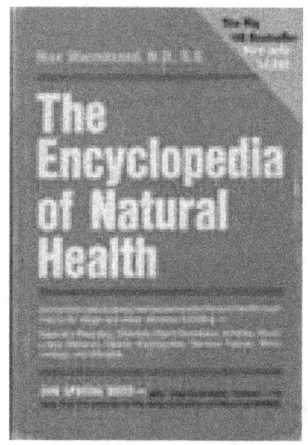

In his book, The Encyclopedia of Natural Health, 1962, Max Warmbrand, N.D., D.O., recommends that, "Remedies containing agar-agar or those manufactured from psyllium seeds or other water-retaining substances are often used to relieve constipation. These remedies act on your colon by absorbing a great deal of water, which is then carried into the large intestine. We do not object too strenuously when these remedies are used to meet a temporary need, but must stress the fact that while they provide relief, they will not correct the underlying weaknesses, which can be done only through the use of good foods, corrective exercises, and a rational way of living."

Agar-agar is seaweed, which is also known by

other names – dai choy goh or kanten. Like psyllium it is mostly soluble fiber. One disadvantage of these fibers is that once they form their bulk in your colon they hold in nutrients that should be absorb through your colon walls

Agar is useful in improving digestion, pulling toxins out of your colon and reducing hemorrhoids.

Ginger

Ginger can stimulate your colon to peristaltic action. It can be used as capsule or as a tea often to keep your bowels moving. In difficult constipation issues, ginger can be used as an enema and at the same time taken as a capsule. It is a gentle colon stimulant.

Ginger is best used in combination with other herbs such as cascara sagrada or rhubarb root. Ginger reduces the discomfort of these strong laxatives and helps to strengthen weak colon walls so peristaltic movement is regained.

Ginger has not been tested to determine its effects on pregnant women. It may not cause a problem, but it is best not to take ginger while pregnant or to consult with your obstetrician before taking it.

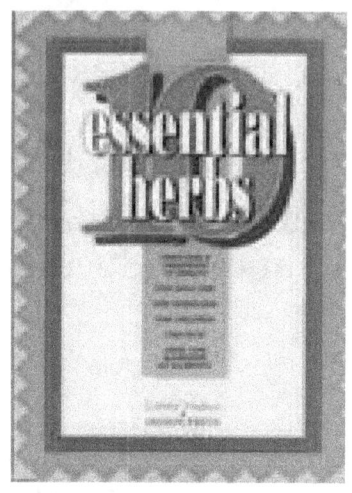

In the book, 10 essential herbs, 1992, Lalitha Thomas gives the ginger combination to relieve constipation. "Chop one oz. fresh Ginger root or one tablespoon of Ginger power if the root is not available Add to this 2 Tablespoons of whole flax seeds Simmer in 2 cups of distilled water for 15 minutes Add honey, unsulfured molasses, or pure maple syrup to taste."

Thomas recommends drinking 1-2 cups of this tea daily and points out that it is safe for children to use but half of this dose.

KYOLIC

Kyolic is a special garlic preparation, which is aged for 20 months in stainless steel tanks.

Kyolic cleanses, soothes, and reduces inflammation throughout your gastrointestinal tract. It is rich in potassium, which is necessary colon wall contraction.

Kyolic is also effective in killing pathogens and bad bacteria that live in your colon and elsewhere in the body. It also binds to heavy metals and other toxins that exist in the blood and colon and sweeps them out of the rectum. Aside from helping in constipation, it is helpful for reducing,

- fungus and other bacteria in your ear
- skin lesions due to bites or insects stings – use liquid form
- arthritis – requires 12 capsules a day
- diabetes – requires 12 capsules a day.

You can buy it in capsule and liquid form. Capsules are easy to take and have no side effects.

Here's how to use it,

- For mild cases of constipation take 2 tablets once or twice a day.
- For moderate cases take 2 tablets three times a day

- For severe cases take 2 tablets five times a day.

Or if you prefer you can take 4-5 Kyolic capsules just before going to bed.

Continuous use of Kyolic is not harmful. It is the allicin in garlic that provides the stimulation to your colon to produce peristaltic movement.

Kyolic can be bought in health food stores or on the Internet, by just typing in **kyolic** into the Google search engine.

Garlic has blood-thinning abilities. Using it with blood thinning drugs, pentoxifylline, NSAID's is potentially dangerous since excessive blood thinning can increase blood-clotting time. Do not use 3 days before any surgical procedure.

Garlic can also cause an allergic reaction or an upset stomach in some people.

Do not use garlic if breast-feeding. Garlic can get into the breast milk giving the baby colic.

Aloe Vera

Menstruating or pregnant women should not use Aloe Vera, in any form, as a laxative.

Aloe Vera is a wonder herb that has been around for thousands of years. It has been used for both external and internal problems – skin rashes, burns, ulcers, internal bleeding. It also promotes bowel movements, which help to relieve constipation. I have found that some people are allergic to Aloe Vera. So if you show a rash or have any other undesirable symptoms, do not use it.

Aloe is an astringent, acts to tighten muscles, and has purgative and laxative action – dispels fecal matter that has collected in your colon. There are many aloe vera gel products to choose from. For best results, choose an aloe gel that is close to that of fresh organic aloe whole leaf gel.

Take two tablespoons of pure aloe vera gel mixed it with apple juice. You can use other types of juices that fit your taste.

If you use aloe juice drink, mix 1/3 of aloe juice

with 2/3 of a juice you like just before bedtime and just on awakening.

Or, if you can handle the taste of the juice, drink a glass of Aloe Vera juice as soon as you wake up and one just before bedtime. This will promote a bowel movement when you wake up.

Aloe Vera can also be taken in capsules. Because aloe can have a strong griping action, it is best to take this herb with a calmative herb such as turmeric. Aloe can also be mixed with powdered fennel seeds. But, you can take aloe as described above and see how you react to it. I know many people who take it without turmeric, and they don't have any side effects.

The best aloe vera is, of course, fresh aloe gel from a leaf. Look for an aloe that has been hand and not machine pressed. When aloe has been machine pressed, it can be contaminated with the yellow sap that is contained in the outer skin of the aloe leaf.

This yellow sap has strong laxative and irritating action in the gastrointestinal tract. A good aloe should not have more than 10 parts per million of yellow sap.

Aloe has been shown to lower blood sugar levels. Diabetics may find a need to decrease medication dosages when using aloe for a longtime. But monitor this with your doctor.

In addition, aloe vera has a cleansing action and restores a healthy balance of the good bacteria in your colon.

Use aloe for 5 days and then rest 2 days. Using aloe on and off like this can help to reduce allergic reactions from long-term use.

Typical recommendations are:

- Aloe gel – 2 tablespoons each day
- Aloe vera juice – 1 quart each day
- Aloe vera concentrate – 5 g up to 3 times each day

Drinking peppermint tea when taking aloe vera capsules can turn aloe vera into a mild natural constipation remedy. You can also mix aloe gel with peppermint tea to form a constipation drink.

Barks and Roots

Black Walnut

The inner bark of the black walnut tree provides a mild and gentle remedy for constipation. Look for black walnut herb in other herbal combinations or make your own combination and add black walnut to your formula.

Black walnut herb is also available as a liquid, tincture, or capsule.

Slippery Elm Inner Bark

Slippery Elm is effective in relieving constipation. It coats and rejuvenates the entire digestion tract by healing any sores or ulcers. It also is high in soluble fiber.

It comes as a capsule or a liquid extract. It is safe and effective for children when used as a tea. You can add a bit of honey to make the kids drink it.

Yellow Dock Root

Yellow Dock is useful in providing a mild to medium laxative action. It acts to stimulate colon peristalsis. It contains Chrysophanic acid and Emodin. Yellow dock root has some antibiotic qualities, is a blood purifier, stimulates the flow of bile, and works on various skin diseases – eczema, hives, and psoriasis.

Look for herbal combinations that have this herb.

Oregon Grape root

It is effective as a laxative and combines well with cascara sagrada and yellow dock root for a more effective laxative mixture. Oregon grape is a gentle liver stimulant that helps to release bile. It is used in all kinds of liver diseases. In addition, Oregon grape helps to detoxify the blood.

Make a tea 2 parts Oregon grape root to ½ part cascara sagrada. Drink 2 oz. at a time, once or twice a day as necessary.

Marshmallow Root

Marshmallow root is gentle laxative and will move fecal matter out of your colon. Use marshmallow root as a tea.

Boil one cup of distilled water. Stir in one heaping teaspoon of marshmallow root. Cover pot and let tea sit for 10-15 minutes. Then, strain the tea and drink it. Take one cup in the morning and one in the evening.

Peppermint Oil

Peppermint is used to soothe the nerves and is useful in relieving constipation when it is due to cramping and anxiety. It contains oils that stimulate the release of bile from the gallbladder. It also improves the function of the cells along your colon. User **peppermint oil as an enteric-coated capsule, so that the capsule does not dissolve in the stomach, but in the small intestine.**

In the small intestine and colon, peppermint relaxes the muscles and promotes the release of gas.

Recommended dose of peppermint oil is 1 capsule three times each day between meals. Use peppermint oil only as recommend on package.

You can also add 2 drops of peppermint oil in an 8 oz. of water and drink after a meal.

Health Alert: Peppermint oil contains menthol, which is poisonous when an overdose is taken. Always follow the recommend manufacturer's dose. If pregnant, do not use the enteric-coated peppermint oil. Do not give peppermint tea or oil to young children.

Golden Seal

Golden seal has a compound, Hydrastine that gives it antiviral and antibiotic properties. It is use to fight off different types of infections internally and externally.

You will see golden seal in some of the herbal formulas for constipation because of its properties to soften fecal matter and to regulate liver functions. It stimulates digestion and bile production, which in turn promotes peristalsis. It also heals the mucosa, your colon wall lining.

Golden seal is considered one of the top 10 herbs in the herbal world.

Do not use Golden seal for more than a week. Do not use it if you are pregnant. Check with your doctor before using it, if you have diabetes, glaucoma, cardiovascular disease, or high blood pressure.

Do not use more golden seal than the recommended dose. In large doses, golden seal may create cardiac arrest or respiratory problems.

Chlorophyll

Chlorophyll is the green substance that occurs in all plant and is one of the most helpful substances you can add to your diet. It helps to strengthen and thicken your colon cell walls. It inhibits the growth of pathogenic bacteria, which can cause various diseases, and feeds the good bacteria.

It detoxifies the cells in your body and colon, which houses an unbelievable amount of toxic matter.

Chlorophyll will help to get your bowels moving by improving your colon function. Use chlorophyll with any of the other methods you use to clear your constipation.

Take 2 capsules of chlorophyll just before meals

The way that I use chlorophyll is by combining 1-2 oz. liquid chlorophyll, juice of one lemon, and 8 oz. of distilled water first thing in the morning. This combination will sit really well in your stomach and you should never have an upset stomachk.

Health Tip: Chlorophyll is considered safe for pregnant and lactating women.

Triphala

Here is a well-known and popular India Ayurvedic herbal product that is available on the Internet and perhaps some India food stores. It is call Triphala. It is effective as a laxative and also has many other benefits such as:

- Improves liver function and digestion
- Reduces high blood pressure and serum cholesterol

Triphala consist of 3 of the tree fruits of Triphala – Harada, Amla, and Bihara.

- Harada is used to treat chronic and acute constipation and anxiety.

- Amla, known for its high vitamin C content and is used to treat body imbalances in the liver, stomach, and intestines. It also fights infections throughout the body.
- Bihara is used to balance and purify excess mucus in the body and especially in the intestines and colon.

Use Triphala for two – three weeks and longer if necessary. This is one combination that you can use for 2-3 months at a time.

Mix ½ teaspoon of Triphala powder with 8 oz. of warm water and drink just before bed time.

Or, Take 2 capsules in the morning and 2 capsules just before you go to bed.

Cabe Jawa

Cabe jawa is a remedy for constipation from Indonesian. It is prepared as follows:

In a glass of 8oz of boiling distilled water with ½ lemon squeezed, add a pinch of ground black pepper and cayenne. Then sip slowly until it is gone.

Herbal Laxative Combination

I have found herbal laxative combinations to be effective in clearing constipation. As with many herbal products, stools can be soft and sometime runny. As you come off these herbal products your stools will normalize. But you can add a bulking product like Psyllium Seed or Hulk to make your stool harder when using herbs. But, better yet you can eat more vegetables and fruits or bran.

Use 1 big Tablespoon of Psyllium seeds with one glass of water 2-3 times each day. Psyllium seeds absorb water and make your stools less runny. In addition, they sweep across your colon walls removing old fecal matter, mucus, and other toxin. This is useful when you have diverticulosis as it helps to pull toxins out of these pockets.

Rhubarb

Rhubarb is a gentle but active laxative when used in small amounts and is considered safe enough for infants. If you use large amounts, it has a strong purgative action. By mixing herbs, you get herbs working together to produce better healing action on the body. Here's a formula that contains rhubarb:

- Rhubarb root -1 part
- Cascara sagrada -1 part
- Ginger -1 part
- Licorice -1 part
- Barberry - 2 parts
- Dandelion - 2 parts

Simmer a cup of this tea and drink just before going to bed.

Here is a herbal tea that is recommended by David Hoffmann, in his book, New Holistic Herbal, 1990

It is a moderate laxative tea combination which provides peristaltic movement by slightly irritating your colon walls and by promoting the release of digestive juice.

Drink this tea just before bedtime.

- Barberry   2 parts
- Boldo or Dandelion   2 parts
- Cascara Sagrda   1 part
- Liquorice   1 part

- Rhubarb Root   1 part
- Ginger or Fennel   1 part

Sometimes, herbs can interact negatively with medications to produce a side effect that can be dangerous.

Some herbs are not properly prepared in standard strength or quality and will not provide you with any benefits of the real herb. As you buy herb products you will become familiar with the companies that produce quality organic products.

Cumin Oil - Children's Remedy

Place a drop of Cumin oil on your finger and let your child smell the oil. Do this just before bedtime. This should promote a bowel movement in the morning.

Using Certain Herbs

Certain herbs such aloe vera, buckthorn, cascara sagrada, frangula, and senna have powerful laxative action. The chemicals called anthraquinones activate this action. Use these herbs as a last resort when trying to clear your constipation.

When these herbs are used too long they can become habit-forming. Use these herbs only if they have been aged. Fresh herbs of this type can irritate your digestive tract and cause vomiting and bloody stools or diarrhea

7: Constipation Nutritional Remedies Doctors Ignore

Minerals

Minerals help the body produce energy and build bones, blood and cells. They are found in the blood and lymph liquid and cell walls. They help in nerve transmission and muscle contractions in your colon. Minerals are used with vitamins and other nutrients to form compounds that are essential for your body's health.

Your body cannot create minerals so you have to get them from the food you eat or through supplements.

Vitamins

Vitamins do not provide energy for the body, they are not found in our tissue, and they do not build cells, but help in converting the food we eat over to nutrients that our body can use.

This means they help enzymes break down our food - protein, fat, and carbohydrates. Your body can make only a few vitamins.

Mineral and Vitamin Supplements

The various minerals and vitamins recommended here should be taken individually or as a multi-mineral complex or as a vitamin complex. Avoid a supplement that contains both vitamins and minerals. There is some loss in the effectiveness of individual vitamins and minerals when they are combined in multiform. Use capsules for best results because capsules are filled with powder. A capsule dissolves quickly and so does the powder.

Some hard, tablet supplements may not dissolve completely in your stomach or intestines and flow into your colon and out your rectum.

Minerals In Fruits and Vegetables

Minerals in produce are the best minerals to take. These minerals are in the form that nature created and is exactly what the body needs. They are electo-magnetically charged and have a life force that is provided by the plant. This life force quickly decreases after the fruit or vegetable has been picked. Therefore, it is always recommended to eat fruits or vegetable soon after they have been picked and not to cook them.

Electrolyte Minerals

It is best to take liquid electrolyte minerals. In this form, minerals have an electrical charge and are ready for use by the body. Electrolyte minerals when placed in the mouth are absorbed quickly though the mouth lining and lining of the gastrointestinal tract as they travel towards colon.

The Next Best Mineral Supplements

If electrolytic minerals are not available, used chelated minerals. These minerals are attached to amino acids making them magnetic, which allow them to flow right through the intestinal walls without having to be digested.

Look for minerals such as,

- Calcium apertate
- Calcium gluconate
- Calcium Citrate

Mineral Absorption

Most minerals are absorbed in the last part of the small intestine and the beginning of the large intestine, your colon. When your colon walls collect layer upon layer of waste, it affects absorption of the minerals you consume. When this happens, your body will be deficient in minerals and your appetite will be larger than normal.

Brewer's Yeast

Brewer's Yeast contains all B vitamins, except B12. It also contains many vitamins, minerals and is high in amino acids.

Brewer's yeast can help to ease, reduce, or clear your constipation. If you can handle the taste, add it to your juices morning and night.

When you first use brewer's yeast, it will create gas in your colon. Brewer's yeast supplements your good bacteria in your colon, increasing its count. This increase in good bacteria activates a battle between the good and bad bacteria creating gas as a by-product. Keep using brewer's yeast until the gas stops. This many take a few weeks but you are doing one of the best things you can do for your health – increasing good bacteria and reducing bad bacteria.

You can improve the benefit of using brewer's yeast by eating cultured yogurt or supplement good bacteria between meals. You want to do this between meals so when you take your supplement your stomach does not put out to much HCl acid, which would kill the supplement.

Health Drug Alert: If you have gout or are taking monoamine oxidase inhibitors do not take brewer's yeast.

MSM

MSM stands for methyl sulfonyl methane. MSM is organic sulfur. It provides many benefits in the body and is widely used as an anti-inflammatory and is especially useful for arthritis pain. MSM is used in all body cells and tissue including joint tissue

MSM in your colon stops or blocks the activity of cholinesterase (ko-li-nes-ter-ace.)

What is cholinesterase?

Our nervous system is composed of a network of nerve cells, which start at the brain and end on all parts of our body. It is nerves that direct muscle contraction or expansion. After the muscle completes its movement, an enzyme **cholinesterase** is released, which stops the muscle from moving again. Without the nerve signal blocking cholinesterase, the muscle would continue to move nonstop.

MSM is useful in clearing up constipation. When I have used MSM, up to 6000-8000mg each day, I have experienced up to 3-4 bowel movements each day. As MSM blocks the activity of cholinesterase, it allows more peristaltic action to occur in your colon. This results in more bowel movements.

Using 2000-4000 mg of MSM, keeps my bowel movements to 2-3 times each day. Of course, for each person the amount will be different.

The action that MSM has in your colon is

useful for older people who have less nerve signals for peristalsis. Cholinesterase stops the few peristalsis signals older people have, thus creating constipation.

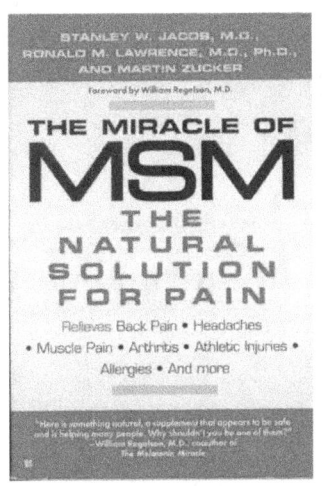

In **S.W. Jacob, M.D., R.M. Lawrence M.D., Ph.D, and M. Zucker book, The Miracle of MSM, 1999, they say,** "As a dietary supplement, MSM offers great potential for anyone with constipation. MSM produces a general "tonic" effect in the bowels and normalizes bowel function, particularly for older individuals. We have given MSM to nursing homes, where constipation is a common problem. The nurses have said that MSM works well for patients, even for individuals not responding to Metamucil or stool softeners."

Rich distributing has good quality products. I have always received good service and quick shipping. I recommend you buy the MSM torpedo tablet. It is a 1000 mg flat oval tablet. This allows you to take 4000-5000 mg of

MSM by only taking 4-5 tablets. They are easy to swallow.

Health Alert: MSM has not been evaluated for effects during pregnancy so it is best not to use it during this time.

Vitamins

The following vitamins help in normalizing and clearing constipation:

Vitamin A

Vitamin A should never be taken by itself. It should be used with other vitamins or taken with food or with fruit snacks.

When taken alone, Vitamin A will putrefy in your colon creating toxic chemicals that may get into your blood.

Vitamin A is an important vitamin, which helps to improve your immunity. Since your colon is an important part of your immune system, it is recommend you eat those foods, which are high in Vitamin A or to use a

Vitamin A supplement. Vitamin A will strengthen your colon.

Vitamin A also helps you absorb protein in your small intestine. Any protein that is not absorbed will move into your colon undigested. In this form and in your colon, this protein decays, producing highly toxic material that can cause serious illness over time.

If you are pregnant or planning to get pregnant, do not take more than 5000 IU each day to avoid birth defects. If you have any liver disease, consult your doctor before taking vitamin A.

B-Vitamins

B-vitamins are needed to feed your colon wall nerves so they can flex and move naturally. Without these vitamins your colon walls cannot move in a natural rhythm.

Eat less sugar and sweets since these foods use up B-vitamins when being digested.

Take **Thiamine** (B1) 100-300 mg each day since it helps to correct constipation by stimulating peristalsis.

Inositol – Helps stimulate your colon walls. Inadequate inositol can be associated with constipation. Drinking too much coffee reduces inositol from the body. Use 100 – 300 mg each day

Folic Acid - If you have constipation and have leg cramps, you may need folic acid. In this case take 400-800 IU of folic acid each day.

Pantothenic acid - 5mg to 3 grams before bed improves the
health of your colon.

Vitamin C

Taking Vitamin C will help to keep you regular. It is a gentle laxative when taken in high doses. When you become constipated, increase your use of Vitamin C. Add 500 mg each day until you reach 5000 mg. At some point you may experience diarrhea. When this happens, just back off on the dose by 500 mg.

When your constipation is cleared go back to your maintenance dose.

Vitamin C in doses greater than 500 mg is not recommended if you have kidney stone, liver disease, or gout.

Vitamin C may increase your absorption of aluminum if you are taking antacids. Take vitamin C two hours before taking antacids to prevent this problem.

Recommend vitamin C dose is 2000 – 3000 mg each day taken with meals. Pregnant women can take up to 500 mg each day.

Minerals - Calcium

Calcium

In your colon, calcium combines with excess bile and decaying fat to form a harmless insoluble soap, which is excreted with your stool. This helps to keep your colon clean.

Most Nutritionists recommend you take 1000 - 1500mg daily of Calcium. Because Calcium can cause constipation, it is necessary to take 500 – 1000 mg of magnesium at the same time you take Calcium.

Health Tip: Space out your intake of calcium over the day. Take only 400 to 600 mg each time. Also take some time-out when taking calcium and other vitamin supplements. In a month, take 2-3 Sundays or Saturdays of from taking vitamins.

Avoid taking calcium carbonate, which will reduce the times you will have a bowel movement. Avoid, also, taking calcium when eating foods that contain oxalates phosphates, or phytates. They tie up calcium and are excreted with the fecal matter

If you are taking a thyroid hormone, beta-blockers, calcium-channel blockers, or an antibiotics, calcium supplements can interfere with adsorption of these drugs.

It is best to take calcium around 2 hours before or after taking these and other drugs.

Avoid taking calcium citrate with aluminum-containing antacids. This combination has been seen to increase your body's absorption of aluminum. Aluminum has been associated with senility and Alzheimer's.

Calcium is safe for pregnant women and they should take an adequate amount of calcium. The best calcium to take is calcium gluconate, orotate or aspartate. The gluconate type is similar to the calcium you get from milk and some vegetables. It is a gentle calcium and is easily absorbed by children and adults with weak digestion.

The foods to eat for good calcium are:

Goat milk, egg yolk, fish, lemons, rhubarb, cheese, skimmed milk, bone broth, seeds, dulse, kelp, greens, nuts, cauliflower, celery, cottage cheese, gelatin preparations, brans,

Mineral - Magnesium

Magnesium, a gentle laxative, helps to prevent constipation by relaxing your colon walls when you are under stress, have anxiety, or have too many worries. It normalizes tension on colon walls allowing for a normal peristaltic action.

Because magnesium attracts water, you can bring in more water into your colon by taking magnesium supplements or by eating foods which are high in magnesium. Water in your colon makes your stools softer and allows your colon to absorb water from your fecal matter if your body needs more water.

How do you know if you are short on magnesium? You will get cramps in your calves at night or so called "Charlie horses." Or, you will feel sore after some mild exercise or activity.

Take 400 mg in the morning and 400 mg in the evening of Magnesium gluconate, or citrate.

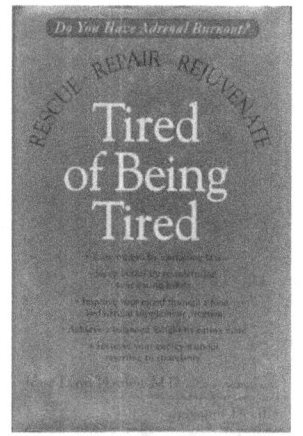

Jesse Lynn Hanley, M.D., in his book call, Tired of Being Tired, 2002, gives another way to take Magnesium to relieve your constipation, "Take at bedtime. Begin with 200 milligrams magnesium oxide or magnesium citrate—you may increase the dosage in 200 milligram increments until your bowels move regularly. The dose for magnesium is individual, so begin low and increase the dosage as needed. Reduce the dosage if you experience loose bowels. Unlike irritating laxatives, magnesium does not create laxative dependency."

If taking hypoglycemic drugs, magnesium may increase absorption of these drugs. It is recommended you consult with your doctor on the effects of magnesium with the type of hypoglycemic drug you are taking.

If taking magnesium, do not take it within 2 hours of taking any kind of drug.

If you have severe kidney or heart disease, you need to avoid magnesium and consult with your doctor on its use.

Magnesium is considered safe for pregnant women.

Foods High in Magnesium

Chlorophyll is high in magnesium and chlorophyll comes in capsules. These are some of the foods that are high in magnesium.

Greens, berries, wheat germ, grains, nuts, cornmeal, apples, apricots, oats, pears, pecans, spinach, tofu, lentils, honey, fish, cabbage, avocados, cashews, peas, prunes, soy milk, chard

Mineral - Iron

Excessive use of iron supplements can cause constipation. To avoid constipation, use between 18 – 30 milligrams of iron.

Food that contain iron are:

Dulse, rice bran, agar, almonds, black cherries, greens, lentils, dried fruits, pinto beans, raisins, rye, sesame seeds, spinach, wheat bran, liquid chlorophyll.

Kelp

Kelp should be taken daily. This provides you with a wide variety of minerals so necessary to rebuild your colon but also to regain good colon function.

Manganese

Manganese works with the B vitamins to strengthen the nerves. It is the nerves in your colon walls that help to activate peristaltic action.

Foods high in manganese are:

Black walnuts, celery, greens, mint, oats, parsley, pineapple, watercress, apples, almonds, beans, blueberries

Pregnant women should not take more than 5mg of manganese each day.

Absorption of manganese is decreased when using antacids or anti-ulcer drugs.

Recommend manganese dose is 5 – 15 mg daily taken with meals.

Potassium and Prunes

Potassium is needed in your colon walls to insure that peristaltic action occurs. Without potassium, colon walls are weak and unable to respond and contract properly when fecal matter needs to be move.

Potassium in your colon wall tissues brings in more oxygen, which is required for good cell function. In addition, potassium creates an alkaline environment inside and outside the cell, which help protect cell walls from germs.

Potassium is a powerful source when it comes to cleaning, feeding and building your colon walls. Removing the thin layer of buildup – harden mucus, dried fecal matter, waste derby, heavy metals - against your colon wall can be accomplished by eating those foods that are high in potassium.

Excess buildup on your colon walls of fecal matter and toxins is a cause of continual constipation. This build up prevents your colon walls from functioning properly.

Potassium is necessary for reducing anxiety and depression. These conditions can affect peristaltic movements of your colon. Lack of it causes muscles and organs to sag and lack tone.

Potassium, also, draws water out of the body. So when potassium is in your colon it attracts water and pulls it into the fecal matter.

To add more potassium to your diet make a drink by,

Pouring hot water over dried prunes and waiting 10 minutes. Then eat the prunes and drink the juice. Or, make a prune smoothie as shown in the Smoothie chapter. Do this on an empty stomach in the morning.

The high concentration of potassium and vitamin A, in prunes, stimulates enzymatic processes. These processes melt down fecal wall wastes and dissolve blockages. They activate peristaltic action to move this waste out your rectum.

The foods that are high in potassium are:

Kale, cabbage, yellow tomatoes, spinach, carrots, broccoli, cucumbers, cauliflower, alfalfa sprouts, goat milk, sesame seeds, wheat germ brewer's yeast, flax seed, grapes, green peppers, pineapple, beets, potatoes with skin Blackstrap molasses

If you have any kidney disease, do not take potassium supplements unless directed by your doctor.
If you are pregnant, take potassium only under a doctor's direction.

If you are on any type of drugs, do not take potassium unless directed by your doctor.

Potassium recommended dose is 1000 – 3000

mg each day taken with meals.

Silicon

Silicon is necessary to firm up and strengthen all the wall structures - blood vessels, colon walls, organ walls, and lymph walls – in the body. It is necessary for nerve impulses to move smoothly from the brain to the vital organs and body.

When you have lost tone in your colon by using laxatives or continual constipation, add silicon to your diet.

One of the highest foods in silicon is rice bran syrup or rice polishing. Other food to consider is:

Oats, barley, kelp, cabbage, apricots, asparagus, beans, nectarines, plums, onions, tomatoes, seeds, nuts, wheat germ, wheat bran, raisins, pumpkin, apples

Recommend dose is 5 – 20 mg each day with meals.

Sodium

Organic sodium, not table salt, is necessary for a number of body functions, including your colon. Organic sodium is only obtained by eating fruits and vegetables.

Sodium keeps the liver and gallbladder working right so the liver does not become enlarged and so the gallbladder does not produce gallstone. In your colon, sodium helps to reduce mucus formation and helps to preserve the proper pH for the good bacteria to flourish.

Without sodium, your body would become acidic and attract all kinds of deadly diseases. Sodium helps to control and neutralize body acids and can keep your body alkaline. An alkaline body is what you need to work towards because disease does not like an alkaline environment. Most people have an acid body.

You can get sodium from, Cow or goat whey, black figs, kale, lentils, okra, black olives Barley, cabbage, carrots, celery, parsley, prunes, sesame seeds, Chickpeas, cheeses, asparagus, beets, coconut, dates, dulse, fish,

Blackstrap Molasses

Blackstrap molasses is a strong laxative. It is high in potassium, calcium, and phosphorous minerals. It also contains some iron, copper, magnesium and B-vitamins.

You can add a teaspoon or tablespoon to your juices. I like adding it to my smoothies on occasion.

Add 1 to 2 tablespoons of molasses a day to hot cereal or mix with warm water and drink it.

Honey

Honey has mild laxative properties. Start by taking a tablespoon three times a day. Add honey to your food, water, drinks or smoothies. Use it the way you like to eat it.

8: Nut and Seed Constipation Remedies You Can Enjoy

Nuts and seeds contain minerals, vitamins, and oils. They can be grounded, chopped, and left whole. In grounded up form, they can be eaten with cereal, fruit, or salads. Or, if you prefer you can eat them whole as a snack.

Nuts and seeds contain a lot of fiber and oils that help to keep you regular and help to relive your constipation.

Flax Seeds

Freshly ground flaxseeds help to soften stools. Take 1 **tablespoon** of flax seeds three times a day. (One tablespoon of flax seeds is equal to 1.5 grams of plant omega-3 fatty acid.) acid.) For severe constipation take 2 tablespoons of flax seeds three times a day. These seeds can be taken whole or grinded up in a coffee grinder.

Grind the seeds and use them immediately to get the benefit of fresh seeds and to avoid their oxidation. Your stomach will not dissolve the whole seed but they will bulk up. Grind them open and you get the benefit of the oil and nutrients that are inside.

You can eat whole flax seeds, but you need to chew them good to break them up. Your stomach will not dissolve whole flax seeds. Chew about a tablespoon in the morning. Then drink 8 oz. of water.

You can grind them up in a grinder and add them to your salads, yogurt, morning cereal, cottage cheese, and smoothies.

It is best not to use them in any cooking recipes. Heat destroys the value of the flax oil and makes it toxic.

I don't recommend you buy ground up flax seeds as listed in the website below. You need to use flax seeds in your drinks or food soon after grinding so they don't lose their nutritive value.

Even though **Nutri Flax**, ground up flax seed, is packaged so the flax seeds don't see light or oxygen, what happens when you open the package? These flax seeds are going to be exposed to oxygen and as time passes they will become oxidized. So it would be important to store Nutri Flax in the refrigerator after it is opened, to minimize its oxidation.

Flax seeds are composed of,

- 41% fat – fifty seven % is omega 3
- 18 % is monosaturated
- 16% is omega 6
- 9% is saturated.
- 20% is protein
- 7% is moisture

It is the high level of omega 3 in flax seeds that make them an essential seed to use in your diet. Flax seed oil helps to decrease the bad effects of omega 6, found high in olive oil. When you eat too much omega 6, you create chronic diseases.

Health Alert: In pregnant women, omega 6, olive oil, blocks the transfer of omega 3 to the baby. This is why a diet should consist of 3 parts omega 6 and 1 part omega 3.

Walnuts and Almonds

Grind equal parts of walnuts and almonds in a coffee grinder. Mix with dark honey into a small ball. Take 3 times a day with two tablespoons of warm water.

Flax Seeds, Seeds, and Nuts

Mix equal parts of flax seeds, almonds, sunflower seeds and sesame seeds. It is O.K. to mix only three of these seeds, if that is all you have.

Grind them in a coffee grinder to a power. You can eat the power or add it to a nondairy smoothie, a juice, or morning cereal. You can also sprinkle it on your evening salad. Use up to 3 tablespoons twice a day.

This mixture will provide you with extra fiber and a batch of minerals.

Drink plenty of water when using ground up seeds.

Flax seeds are astringent and have laxative action. They are good for mild or moderate symptoms of constipation.

Using an excess of flax seed can contribute to the backup in your colon. Flax seeds also have small traces of prussic acid, which is toxic in large amounts. But, it would take a lot of flax seeds to reach the toxic level.

Place between 1 teaspoon to 1 tablespoon of flax seed in 8 oz. of warm water and let it sit for one hour. Then just before going to bed, drink the 8 oz. After drinking this glass of flax seeds, drink another 4-8oz of water.

Flax Seed and Apple Cider Vinegar

Boil 1 ½ cup of distilled water.

Add 1 tablespoon of flax seed and continue boiling the water for 10 minutes – tea will become jelly like.
After this cools down add 1 teaspoon of apple cider vinegar.

Drink cup of this combination in the morning and until you get good daily bowel movement.

Flax seed contains the essential oil omega 3. Essential oil means without this oil you cannot live. If you lack this oil in your diet you will be prone to disease.

Apple cider vinegar (ACV) is another extremely important food you should include in your daily eating. ACV is high in various minerals and in particular potassium

Flax Seeds and Oats

To get your bowels moving again, prepare the following mixture.

Mix 1 tablespoon of flax seed and 1 tablespoon of oat bran into a glass of distilled water. Let it sit overnight. First thing in the morning, take 2 tablespoons. Wait half an hour before eating anything. Do this every morning until your bowels start moving

Flax Seed Oil

Our body does not make omega 3 oil and we need to get it in our diet.

For constipation, mix one tablespoon of flax seed oil with goat or cow yogurt. Add a little honey if you like. Take this mixture right about ½ hour before bedtime.

Do not heat flax seed oil and keep it refrigerated. Heating it may cause some cancer causing compounds.

Fenugreek Seeds

Use 1-2 teaspoons with juice or water, 2-3 times each day. This seed will bulk up like the psyllium seed so drink plenty of water during the day.

Fenugreek can lower blood sugar levels, so check with your doctor before using it with diabetic drugs.

Pregnant women should not use fenugreek because of its ability to stimulate contractions.

Psyllium, Flax, Fenugreek Seed Combination

Combine flax seeds, fenugreek seeds, and Psyllium seeds. Use 3 tablespoons of this combination each day..

Pumpkin seeds

Pumpkin seeds are a mild laxative, which can activate peristalsis. Eat seeds that are still in the shell throughout the day. You can also grind them up and add them to your salads or smoothies.

Black Sesame Seeds

For chronic constipation, **Maoshing Ni, Ph.D., C.A. and Cathy McNease, B.S., M.H. in their book, The TAO of Nutrition,1987, recommend using black sesame seeds.**

- Grind black sesame seeds into a meal by using a small coffee grinder.

- Mix with dark honey into a small ball.
- Eat one three time a day dipped in rice wine.

Black sesame seeds also provide nutrition and action on the liver, intestines, kidney, and blood.

You can also prepare a **sesame seeds soup** with brown rice.
- Soak 10 parts of sesame seeds with 1 part brown rice in distilled water.

- After they are soft, about an hour, pour out the water grind them in a small food grinder to produce liquid. Strain the remaining liquid to remove coarse particles.

- Dilute liquid with distilled water and add some honey.
- Cook on low heat until liquid becomes syrupy.

Drink around two cups to relieve constipation within hour or so.

Peas and brown sesame seeds – help to lubricate the intestinal walls. This makes it easier for fecal matter to move through your colon.

Sunflower seeds

Sunflower seeds promote regularity. Use them raw shelled and unsalted every day. They contain omega-6 fatty acid just like olive oil. You can use them grounded and add them to your morning smoothie, 1-2 teaspoons, or to your homemade salad dressing

- Add them to your salad

- Add them to your morning cereal

Here's a sunflower drink you can make.

Take 1-2 tablespoons of sunflower seeds. Grind them in a coffee grinder. Add them to a cup of boiling water. Sweeten this mixture with honey, maple syrup, or blackstrap molasses. Drink this combination morning and night to help you with you constipation.

Coconuts

Coconuts can relieve your constipation. Eat fresh coconut two-time a day, once in the morning and in the evening. Coconut water is high in various minerals and the meat are high in good fatty acids.

9: How to Use Fiber For Constipation

What is Fiber?

Fiber is a carbohydrate that comes from the cell walls and structure of plants, grains, legumes, fruits, and vegetables. Most processed or junk food has little fiber, which is removed during processing.

Most people eat around 7-12 grams of fiber each day. You should be eating from 25 – 45 grams each day to prevent serious illnesses in your body.

A diet with 40 grams of fiber provides protection and prevention against diseases such as kidney stones, varicose veins, obesity, heart disease, appendicitis, colon disease, diabetes, appendicitis, diverticulosis, and many others.

When you eat fiber, it passes into your colon without getting digested in the small intestine.

The good bacteria will use some of it as food, which makes them stronger and able to multiply.

Eating fiber reduces your fecal matter transit time from 3 days to 1 1/ 2 - 2days.

All processed foods, such as white flour products, have little or no fiber. Fiber is removed when various natural flours or grains are processed to make junk food. During this processing, nutrients, vitamins, and minerals are also removed. Only plant foods and lightly processed grains have fiber of varying amounts

Fiber, bulk, or roughage, is one of the main nutrients you need to eat daily to relieve and prevent constipation and prevent many other diseases. Fiber is a nondigestible, complex carbohydrate. Most fiber is fermented in your colon and provides some energy for the body.

Seaweed Fiber

Agar and alginate come from seaweed and are indigestible. They are used in gelatinous foods to make desserts. Alginate is especially useful since it can bind to harmful metals such as lead, arsenic, mercury, and cadmium and move them out of your body through your stools.

Eating Fiber

As you can see fiber is a critical nutrient for your colon and overall health. You need to eat equal amounts of insoluble and soluble fiber. Most people only eat around 10 grams or less of fiber each day. The amount you need to eat is around 25 – 45 grams. This is a lot of fiber and you will need to introduce it slowly into your diet. You may experience gas when you eat more fiber.

If you have any serious gastrointestinal illnesses, check with your doctor before adding more fiber to your diet.

One other major benefit of fiber is that, **fiber stimulates pancreatic secretions - enzymes and bicarbonates -which help you to digest your food better and prevents undigested protein from reaching your colon.**

When you are constipated, your fecal matter remains in contact with your colon walls longer. Undigested protein that is embedded in the fecal matter starts to decomposes and putrefies. This undigested protein and putrid matter serve to feed bad bacteria and changes your colon environment into a toxic generator.

If you have not been eating a lot of fiber in the form of vegetable, fruits and grains, you need to add these foods to your eating habits slowly so your body gets use to more fiber.

The more fiber you eat the more vitamins and minerals are lost and eliminated in your stools. What this means, is you need to compensate for this lost by eating more nutritious foods and or by using supplements.

Provide yourself with natural forms of fiber, such as vegetables, fruits, and legumes. Stay away from the supplemental forms of fiber such as, powders or pills that may help in relieving constipation but do little to provide you with other nutrients those natural forms of fiber provide.

Supplemental fiber granules, powders, or pills can become addictive.

Limit your use of fiber that comes from grains. I know you have been told you need to eat a lot of bran, whole wheat products, cereals, oats, oatmeal, buckwheat, unprocessed bran, rice bran, and so on.

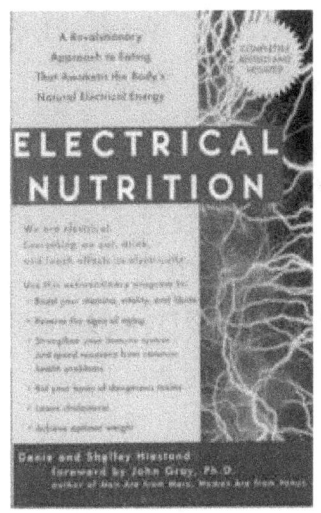

In their recent book, 2001, *Electrical Nutrition*, **Denie and Shelley Hiestand** points out that our digestive system was not designed to process grains. When we eat food, our digestive system was designed to ferment food to break them down and make their nutrients available for our bodies. The Hiestand's continue,

"Our digestive tract, like that of the grazing animals, is almost completely unable to ferment a seed-head (grain), whether it is whole or ground up as in flour...when we try to eat grain, the innate frequency of the seed-head can only go into storage—in other words, lay downcellulite...

This is why in agriculture to fatten up the hog or cattle, we feed them grain. Likewise, if you want to fatten up, eat grains... they take the most energy to digest, and we get little or nothing from it except large thighs, butts, and bellies. REMEMBER THE OLD FARM SAYING GRAINS FOR GAIN, PROTEIN FOR PRODUCTION. From an electrical nutrition perspective, modern grains could well be considered toxic."

Limit the use of grains to get your fiber. Make more use of vegetables, fruits, and legumes to get fiber. However, when trying to clear constipation, fiber from bran can be used for a limited time.

Eating Bran

Eating bran is one of the quickest and best ways to increase your fiber. It will increase the weight and size of your stools more than the fiber contained in fruits or vegetables. Bran is the outer husk of the grain – wheat, corn, rice, oat – which is indigestible.

It does not irritate the lining of the stomach, small intestine or your colon. It is not a laxative but promotes the movement fecal matter through your colon in a natural way. Unlike drugstore laxatives or other naturally strong laxatives, bran does not quickly purge out all the contents in your colon.

Use one or two heaping tablespoon of bran in your morning cereal, in your baking, and in your smoothies.

Health Alert: When using bran, make sure you drink plenty of water during the day to keep your stools soft.

Here are some other ways to use bran. You can add them to,

- baked breads, muffins and other baked goods
- breaded mixes
- hamburger meat
- juices
- pancake or waffle mix
- salads
- scramble eggs
- soups
- soups
- stuffing
- vegetarian burger mix
- yogurt

When you put bran in juices or anything that is all liquid just eat it with a spoon.

How much bran should you take for good bowel regularity? Each person is different. You need to experiment. Start with two teaspoons each day and work towards 10 teaspoons a day or until you have bowel movements without effort or straining.

There are four basic bran products – wheat, corn, oat, and rice. They all provide a solid source of fiber in varying amounts. Make sure the bran you use is 100% unprocessed bran.

Use bran for a few weeks to get your bowel movements back to normal. Eating bran should get your bowels moving in a few days or less.

Once your bowels are back to normal, back off from using a lot of bran and depend more on fiber from eating more fruits, vegetables, nuts, and seeds.

There are many new products, which use bran added to other nutrients or powders. Although these can be useful, use them for a limit time. Chapter21 lists some of these products.

Wheat Bran

Many people use wheat bran to get more fiber in their diet. This was something that was encouraged in the past. But now you should limit or reduce the use of bran as a way to get more fiber in your diet.

Wheat bran is not the best bran to use but can be used in combination with oat, rice, or corn bran, which is better.

Wheat bran consists mainly of insoluble fiber. It consists of cellulose, hemi-cellulose, lignin, pectin, and pentosans. It absorbs plenty of water making the stools bulky and soft, which allows them to move through your colon easily. Bulky fiber stools help to scrub your colon walls to keep them clean of mucus and toxic build up.

There are many more nutritious ways to add fiber to your diet. Eating any bran requires drinking plenty of water throughout the day otherwise it can cause constipation.

When eating bran in any form, cereal, pancakes, or muffins, always drink extra water during the day. Bran absorbs water and becomes larger. Use water to help move it easily through your colon.

Young children should not eat wheat or rice bran. Eating bran requires drinking plenty of water throughout the day. Eating too much bran can cause the fecal matter to become too bulky and can cause constipation instead of relieving it.

Bran contains a high level of phytates, which interferes with absorption of calcium, zinc, iron and copper. For this reason use a maximum of 1/3 of a cup of bran each day for yourself and for children use 1/6 of a cup. Excess use of wheat bran would require taking calcium, zinc, iron and copper supplements.

Bran is also high in B-vitamins and consists of around 21% protein.

Children should not eat as much fiber as adults. Children should eat oat cereal, whole grain cereals, fruits and vegetables.

Corn Bran

Corn bran has even more fiber than wheat bran by 40%. So, corn bran is excellent for prevent constipation. Both corn bran and wheat bran should be used in moderation and not used as the main ingredient in trying to prevent constipation.

Oat Bran

Oat bran has both soluble and insoluble fiber, which make its better to use than wheat bran. However, it does have less insoluble fiber than wheat and rice bran. It can be found with relatively little processing which helps to maintain its high quality of protein, carbohydrates and vitamins.

Keep away of commercially made oat, wheat or other type of bran muffins since they contain a lot of fat, sugar and other additives that are unhealthy for you.

Rice Bran

For preventing constipation, rice bran is better than wheat bran.

In their book called High Speed Healing, 1991, the editor of Prevention Magazine Health Books, said that, "You may see a dramatic improvement in your fight against constipation by using rice bran-instead of wheat – to

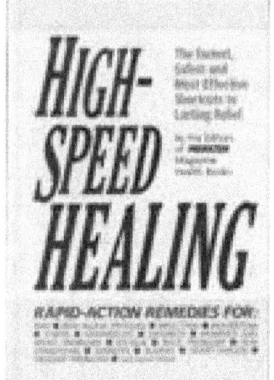

increase the size and frequency of your stools. One European study says that rice beats the living chaff out off wheat when it comes to fecal output and frequency of bowel movements."

Health Tip: Do not take your calcium supplement with bran cereals since fiber can interfere with calcium absorption.

Do not use cereal with bran in it. This bran has been processed and loses some of its fiber content. Use the bran sold as coarse granules. Add it to your morning cereals, smoothies, shakes, cottage cheese, yogurt, or other dishes.

Soy Bran

Soy bran is not a recommend source of bran. Despite the popularity of soy there are some effects of soy that are not healthy. Soy is a high source of lignin fiber and other chemicals, which can block absorption of:

- minerals
- protein
- trypsin

Soy also has a high-level of phytoestrogens, which help to reduce the harmful effects of excess estrogen but soy products are not good for children who do not need a high-level phytoestrogens.

Soy used fermented – miso or tempeh –is an excellent food but still have traces of chemicals that block the body's absorption of certain minerals. Tofu can be used but should be eaten with foods high in minerals.

Despite the efforts of the soy industry to remove some of the chemicals that are not good for human consumption, there are still traces of these chemicals in soy milk and tofu.

Sources of Insoluble Fiber

- Bananas
- Broccoli
- Brown rice
- Brussels sprouts
- Cauliflower

- Cabbage
- Corn
- Lentils
- Potatoes
- Spinach wheat germ
- Whole wheat bread
- Whole wheat crackers

Sources of Soluble Fiber

Oranges, grapefruit, nectarines, peaches, tangerines, apples, berries, apricots, bananas, figs, prunes

Zucchini, turnips, okra, cabbage, peas, sweet potatoes, Carrots, celery, broccoli, cauliflower, corn, eggplant, okra, Zucchini, greens Barley, chickpeas, split peas, pinto beans, kidney beans, navy beans, potatoes

If you have a colon disease, check with your doctor before including more fiber in your diet.

Remember each one of us needs a different amount of fiber. You decide how much fiber you should include in your diet. Just make sure it is more than 30 gm. each day.

If you are pregnant or lactating, eating fiber is considered safe.

Digestive Enzymes

Be carefully when using HCL supplements. If your stomach is normal, additional acid can cause stomach ulcers or irritate your stomach lining.

Digestion and assimilation of food starts in the mouth. As your food travels into your stomach, Hydrochloric Acid, HCL, works on the protein and in your small intestine digestive enzymes complete the breakdown your food.

Your stomach produces HCL, whenever you eat protein, fat, or are stressed. When you overeat or eat too frequently, your stomach cannot produce enough HCL to digest the protein or fat you have eaten. This results in incomplete protein digestion, bloating, or gas.

Secreting good levels of HCL stimulates the pancreas to release adequate levels of digestive enzymes, which continue digestion of protein, fats and carbohydrates in the small intestine.

Eating a healthy diet, less food or protein at a sitting, and reducing stress can help return your HCL levels to normal.

Anyone with digestive problems should take digestive enzyme supplements. The older you get the more important it is to take this supplement. As you age, secretions from various organs start to diminish and your body is deprived of these needed secretions.

Take digestive enzymes 30-45 minutes before meals to improve you digestion. Taking digestive enzymes between meals can help with food allergies.

HCL supplements can be obtained as betaine hydrocholoride. It can be found as a single supplement or in combination with other digestive enzymes.

If you have ulcers of any kind, do not use digestive enzymes.

There are various digestion enzymes you can use. Visit a health food store to find one that you like.

Bromelain

Drug Health Alert: Bromelain thin blood, so it is best not to take it when using the blood thinning drugs Coumadin and warfarin. If you get any allergic reactions to Bromelain, stop using it right away.

Bromelain also has the ability to increase the effectiveness of any antibiotics you take.

Bromelain is found in pineapples and is useful in digesting protein. It has other benefits such as reducing inflammation and platelet aggregation and clot formation.

Bromelain is useful when there is a decrease in the enzymes produced by the pancreas.

There are some people that are allergic to pineapples so they should not take Bromelain. As a digestive aid use Bromelain with meals. As an anti-inflammation nutrient use it between meals.

Recommended dose is 1400 – 1800 MCU each day.

If you are pregnant, it is considered safe to use

Bromelain.

Papain

Papain, a mild digestive enzyme, is found in papayas and helps in protein digestion.

Amylase, Proteases and Lipases

Amylases, proteases, and lipases are the major group of digestive enzymes, which are secreted by the pancreas. Amylase digests carbohydrates, protease digest protein, and lipase digests fats. These enzymes are available in capsules and should be taken just before you eat.

It is best to use enteric enzymes, which are capable of reaching the small intestine where they are needed. These enzymes are coated so they can pass through your stomach HCL without getting destroyed.

Good Bacteria

Health Drug Alert: If you are taking antibiotics, you need to take a "good bacteria" supplement. Antibiotics will kill many of the bad and good bacteria in your colon allowing the bad bacteria to become more dominant. When this happens, you are more susceptible to creating an in-balance in your colon and creating diarrhea.

Acidophilus is a good bacteria. It must be the dominant bacteria in your colon; otherwise, you will be susceptible to many colon problems including constipation.

How can you bring good bacteria like acidophilus into your colon. The stomach acids and the high alkaline environment of the small intestine prevent any reasonable amount of acidophilus to reach your colon. And, any acidophilus that does reach your colon will most likely be attacked and destroyed by the bad bacteria. If your colon is toxic and alkaline, this furthers the chances the acidophilus will be destroyed in your colon.

It is best to first feed your good bacteria with milk whey as described elsewhere so the exist good bacteria can multiple. Once this is done and you reestablish a high-level of good bacteria in your colon, then take acidophilus and other good bacteria by,

- Taking 2-3 **regular** capsules of good

bacteria between meals with distilled water so to not activate the high levels of destructive stomach acid.

- Taking 2-3 **enteric** capsules of good bacteria so the good bacteria by passes the stomach acids and opens in the small intestine.

Barley

Eating muffins or other breads made from barley flakes or flour has shown to clear up constipation. Eat around 3 muffins each day. Make sure you drink plenty of water during the day. Barley has been found to reducing heart, cancer, and digestive problems

Beans

All kinds of bean and peas can help you erase your constipation and prevent it. Beans have are high in fiber and will make your stool softer and increase its stool size. Beans also stimulate the good bacteria in your colon by providing short chain fatty acids, which they use for food.

Here's how to use beans for constipation.

Cooking - Clean beans with distilled water to remove dirt and small rocks. Soak beans for 4-8 hours. Dump water and place beans into a crock pot. Set the pot to low and add some garlic cloves, onions and chili powder. At the low setting, the beans will cook under 112 degrees F. At this temperature the enzymes in the beans will not be destroyed. These cooked beans will be considered live food. Cook the beans for around 8 hours or until soft and eatable.

Eat one half cup to one cup of beans daily to break up constipation. The fiber available in one of cup of different types of beans is:

- Black eye beans 7.4 grams
- peas, canned 5.4 grams
- Kidney beans 5.0 grams
- Pinto beans 4.6 grams
- Navy beans 4.6 grams
- Lentils 1.7 grams

A Lentils Soup Remedy

Here a soup recipe that will relieve your constipation. Cook lentils and make a soup adding the following:

- Add cooked brown rice
- Add carrots, celery, onions, garlic
- Add a tablespoon of lecithin when adding Prune Juice, Applesauce, and Oat Bran

Mix, in a bowl, equal amounts of,

- Prune juice
- Applesauce
- Oat bran or any other bran
- Six ground up almond
- A squeeze of lemon

Make the consistency to your liking.

Take 3 tablespoons or more each day. Best time is morning, noon and night.

Agar-Agar

Agar is a type of seaweed that can be used to help relieve constipation in 2-8 day if you use it every day. Boil it in water to dissolve it and form a jelly. Flavor it with a juice, a fruit puree, and honey or any other type of flavoring that appeal to you.

Saltwater Cleansing

Saltwater has a fast action in clearing out your colon. If you need to clear your constipation fast this is the method to use. Do not use this method often since it purges everything out of your colon good or bad. After using this method follow it with a week or two of good bacteria supplements.

Salt has a softening effect on hard fecal matter in your colon and helps to lubricate your colon walls. Limit your salt intake if you have high blood pressure or edema. Salt in excess has a damaging effect on the blood. However, seaweeds, herbs, vegetables that contain sodium and other mineral salts are not harmful to the body.

It is best to use sea salt for this cleansing. Sea salt has many minerals that are beneficial to your health. Only use regular salt if cannot get sea salt.

Add two teaspoons of sea salt to a glass of warm distilled water. Drink on an empty stomach. Drink first thing in the morning. You should have a bowel movement within one hour.

Do not use this method if you have edema or hypertension

Bentonite

Bentonite is a natural clay mineral that comes from volcanic ash that has eventually become clay. This clay has special properties that enable it to clean out your colon of toxic matter. It is high in sodium and this gives it electrical properties that help bind toxic matter to its atomic structure.

Bentonite is useful in assisting fruits and vegetables to clean out your colon and makes it an area more livable for good bacteria. It also is good for reducing constipation.

Choose only high purity bentonite, which contains high levels of sodium and low levels of calcium. Great Plains Bentonite makes one such product.

10: The Real Cause of Constipation

Causes of constipation

Your colon is designed to move undigested matter and various bodily wastes through its tract and out the rectum. It does this naturally only when this matter and waste have bulk or fiber. It is this bulk or fiber that pushes against your colon walls and triggers peristaltic action. You can only get this bulk when you eat plenty of fruits, vegetables, and grains that have a combination of soluble and nonsoluble fiber.

Meat, fish, and dairy products have little or no fiber. In your colon these foods do not move easily and remain too long in your colon.

Constipation habits come from unnatural living Constipation is a complex symptom that is caused by many conditions that have amassed in the body and cause your colon to malfunction.

Constipation can be caused by a physical

weakness due to surgery, inactivity, or deformities, which were inherited or acquired through injury or surgery. Constipation cause by these conditions can be improved by using natural nutrients and alternative methods. However, it is more difficult to help this type constipation since the physical conditions have to be improved.

The continual use of medications or drugs of any sort can cause constipation. It can be cause by the excess use of laxatives. It can be continual use of certain minerals or vitamins.

Psychological constipation

Constipation is also related to psychological and emotion issues. Anxiety will cause the nerves, wall tissue and muscles in your colon to tense up. If you have a personality that holds feeling or thoughts inside you and do not discuss them with those people you should, you will mostly likely have continual constipation.

If you have stresses and anxieties in your life, constipation can be a result. Anxiety can also overwork the Adrenal gland making it output cortisol. Overtime, because cortisol is toxic to the brain, cortisol will damage and kill brain cells, which can lead to premature old age and Alzheimer's. You will also feel tired and run down when you over stress your Adrenal.

Sometimes constipation can suddenly appear when changes in normal living habits and stressful conditions have occurred – flying out of your time zone, having personal confrontations at work or within the family.

Infrequent bouts with constipation are really nothing to worry about and can be corrected with many of the suggestions listed in this e-book

The main cause of constipation is the continual eating of processed foods, which have little food value or fiber and are packed with poison additives. This results in colon wall weakness where fecal matter cannot even be push out of the rectum.

Eating food with little or no fiber creates fecal matter that is mushy or hard and compacted. Mushy or compact fecal matter is hard to move along your colon and your colon walls tire after many peristaltic movements. After a time, your colon walls stop trying and you end up with constipation.

Constipation is a body condition you have created by improper living choices, which you can change. It is sometimes an easy symptom to eliminate and at other time difficult to deal with.   It occurs from a complex of many things. Like so many other body conditions or illnesses, it is a result of:

- Absorbing too many toxins into the body
- Anxiety and depression
- Being bedridden
- Having colitis, or spastic colon.
- Having diabetes
- Having diseases of the anus or rectum such as Having tumors, diverticulosis
- Drinking coffee
- Drinking milk
- Drinking sodas
- Drinking tea
- Eating excess protein
- Eating food that doesn't have fiber
- Eating processed foods
- Eating sugars
- Eating too much food at one sitting
- Excess exposure to organophosphate

insecticides
- Excess use iron supplements
- Excess use of enemas
- Excess use of seasonings
- Excessive Calcium in the body
- Fatigue
- Food sensitivities
- High fever – colon accumulates heat and hardens stools
- Hypothyroidism, Low levels of thyroid hormone IBS
- Kidney failure
- Lack of good bacteria
- Mineral Deficiency
- Nerve disorders of your bowel
- Not chewing food completely
- Not drinking enough water
- Not enough exercise
- Older people
- Overeating
- Overuse of laxatives
- Overdose of Vitamin D
- Parasites
- Poor digestion
- Postponing a bowel movement
- Pregnancy
- Premenstrual tension

- Spinal injuries – people with these injuries can have damage to the nerves that regulate bowel moments
- Toxic liver
- Use of prescription drugs
- Various diseases

Constipation can be a symptom of the start of a disease or illness. Do not take OTC laxatives, which will mask the illness that eventually has to be dealt with.

Absorbing too many toxins

Taking in too many toxins – pesticides, insecticides, heavy metals, food additives, and air pollution - from various sources can create constipation. Each of these toxins and chemicals can have different reaction in your colon so your colon does not function properly.

Anxiety and Depression

Sometimes, people who have excessive repressed feeling, which is the cause of anxiety and depression, keep thoughts and behaviors inside themselves. This personality characteristic can be associated with constipation.

By holding feelings to yourself, your mind will reflect your thoughts throughout your body and hold on to your fecal matter. Holding in your feelings puts tension in your colon muscles leading to constipation.

Drinking Coffee and Tea

Note although coffee can be a laxative; caffeine can also contribute to constipation in some people.

Tea

Drinking up to 68 oz. of tea each day is known to cause constipation.

Drinking Sodas

Drinking sodas is probably one of the most harmful habits. In recent clinical studies, it was found to interfere with life span. It contains excess sugar and can interfere with your digestion and continual use can result in insulin spikes. When food is not digested properly, it leads to undigested food, reaching your colon.

Eating excess protein

Protein from meat has no fiber. It is high in saturated fat. Both of these characteristics lead to constipation. Without fiber it is difficult for meat to move through your colon. Excess saturated fat, in your colon, attracts and binds minerals, which are moved out in your stools. These minerals are necessary for your body and colon's health and are normally reabsorbed through your colon wall.

Eating Processed Foods

Constipation is caused by eating white flour, sugar, bread, cheese, and processed foods. It is these foods that weaken the spleen, which is responsible for passing energy to your colon to function properly.

It helps to eat whole bran or whole-wheat products to eliminate constipation, but straight bran stresses the body since the body is not eating a balanced food Bran is a partial food, it is part of the wheat.

Eating Sugars

Sugar is a processed food that has no nutrient value and has no fiber. Using it over a longtime eventually is a cause of constipation.

Excess Iron Supplement

Constipation is associated with taking excessive iron supplements. However, there are some studies that suggest that this is not the case. If you are taking iron supplements and constipated, you can always experiment by reducing your intake to see if your constipation is relieved.

When under a doctor's care, Always check with your doctor before changing iron doses.

I always recommend you take your mineral supplements when you have a meal and this includes iron supplements.

Excess use of enemas

Using too many enemas is like overusing laxatives. Your colon becomes lazy and becomes dependent on the enemas to move the fecal matter out the rectum.

Excess use of seasonings

Using an excess use of pepper, salt, and condiments can lead to constipation. Limit your use of these seasoning. Overtime decrease the amount of salt and pepper you use to season your food. Learn how to use herbs to season your food.

When you eat too much salt, more water is absorbed through your colon walls, leaving your fecal matter with less than 80% water. When this happens your fecal matter becomes dry and hard, making it difficult for you to have a bowel movement.

When you do not have enough salt in the foods you eat, less water is pulled through your colon walls. This leaves your fecal matter with excess water. Your fecal matter will not have much form and your stools will be watery.

You don't have to add salt to your food to get the right amount of sodium into your colon. The salt you really need is organic salt, which you get from eating fruits and vegetable.

Excessive Calcium in the body

Taking an excess of calcium can weaken colon muscles and cause constipation. What is an excess of calcium? A recommended level for calcium is around 1000-1500 mg each day. Calcium must also be balanced with other minerals especially magnesium.

Calcium should never be taken as a single supplement but should be taken in combination with other minerals and taken with meals.

Mineral Deficiency

When your body is deficient in minerals, you will have an acid body that will not function well. Your colon typically recycles ionic minerals by pulling them out of the fecal matter, moving them through your colon wall, and transferring them into the bloodstream.

You need minerals to neutralize the excess acids in your small intestine, colon and throughout your body. Without a constant supply of minerals, your colon will not function like it should.

Overeating

If you overeat, your body may not be able to digest all of this food. Undigested food is not be absorbed in the small intestine and will move into your colon. This undigested food is difficult to move through your colon and can cause constipation. This slow moving undigested food will decay, create gas, and produce a toxic colon.

Large amounts of slow moving fecal matter in your colon and the gas produced will enlarge your colon. Repeated enlargement of your colon will weaken your colon walls and lead to less peristaltic action.

Not drinking enough water

One of the functions of your colon is to remove water from fecal matter as it passes through your colon. This prevents your body from eliminating too much water through your stools and becoming dehydrated. The removed water is used in your blood and lymph liquid.

When you do not drink enough water, fecal matter will not move through your colon quickly. This gives your colon walls more time to remove water from your fecal matter. This in turn causes your fecal matter to become hard and dry. When fecal matter gets hard, it becomes difficult to move through your colon. The longer it stays in your colon, the harder it gets. Peristaltic action will move it slowly and as more fecal matter enters your colon from other meals you will soon be constipated.

Under normal conditions, your body alerts you to when you need to drink water by making you feel thirsty. This should be your guide to how much water to drink. The problem arises when you ignore this thirst and your body becomes dehydrated.

This is why it is recommended you keep track of how much water you drink, 32 oz. minimum. However don't force yourself to drink more water. But do have water available so when you feel thirsty you can drink right away.

If you have pain in the lower left part of your abdomen because of constipation, drinking water should relieve this pain.

Not enough exercise

In her booklet, Dietary Fiber, 1988, Shirley S. Lorenzni, Ph.D, states,

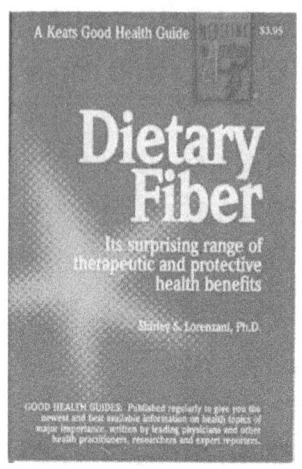

"Inactivity contributes to constipation. You may have noticed this during a period of bed rest or while you are traveling. Some scientists believe that lack of physical exercise, not old age, causes constipation in the elderly. A recent study in African revealed a definite connection between exercise and fecal output"

Older People

As you age, you are more likely to have constipation. As you get older, the walls of your intestines and colon weaken and loose tone. This makes it more difficult to have good strong wall movements, which are necessary to move chime and fecal matter through your intestines and colon.

Colon weakens when you don't supply the right minerals to your colon walls. Plenty of potassium is needed to make your colon walls flex. Potassium is obtained from both fruits and vegetables.

Tone is lost when you don't exercise and eat

the right foods. Exercise forces your stomach muscles to contract and extend. This movement strengthens your intestinal and colon walls and at the same time helps to push fecal matter in your colon towards your rectum.

Cells that secrete water along the intestinal walls decrease, as you get older. Overtime less water is secreted and absorbed by the fecal matter making them harder. This condition makes the fecal matter difficult to move along your colon.

Overuse of laxatives

Using laxatives, damages nerves inside your colon walls. When used excessively, you can become dependent on them. Drugs store laxatives can create the condition you are trying to eliminate – constipation. Use them sparingly or consult a doctor before using them.

Overdose of Vitamin D

Taking an excess of vitamin D can cause constipation. This does not happen to often since most people produce enough vitamin D by being out in the sun. The problem can arise for children and older people who are confined indoors and need to take vitamin D supplements.

Parasites

Most parasites that we absorb from outside our body live in your colon. Of course we also see them in our blood, lymph liquid, organs and even on our skin. These parasites attach themselves to your colon walls and cause many irritating symptom like diarrhea, constipation, flatulence, headaches, and poor memory. They can also cause more serious problems such as holes in your colon wall. When this happen fecal matter can cross your colon wall, get into your blood, and cause allergic reactions.

Don't think you don't have parasites. This would be a big mistake. Most everyone has some sort of parasites in their body.

In her book, Parasites – THE ENEMY WITHIN, Hanna Kroeger, 1991-2001, says, "Here are some dietary suggestions. A diet high in carbohydrates and low in protein has been found to make parasitic infections worse. When the body is in an alkaline condition the parasitic infection sets in. It is best to keep the diet slightly acidic both as a preventive measure and when treating the infection. Foods that help keep the intestines acidic are apple cider vinegar and cranberry juice."

Parasite waste and excretions are toxic to your body and make your colon pH more alkaline. You need your colon to be slightly acidic. This makes your colon more livable for your good bacteria.

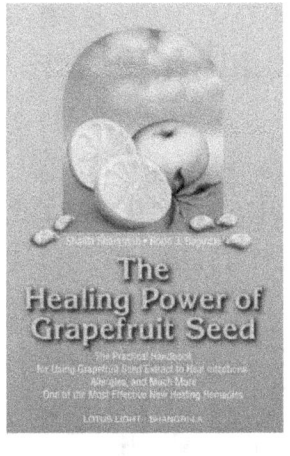

In their book, The Healing power of Grapefruit Seed, 1997, Shalila Sharamon and Bodo J. Baginski summarized the importance of using grapefruit seed extract, "After we have seen how easily pathogens - whether they are bacteria, viruses, fungi, or parasites – get into our body and how much havoc they can wreak, the question may arise: "Wouldn't it be smart to take a few drops of grapefruit seed extract every day as a preventative against the uninvited guests? Since it is non-toxic, it can't do any harm but will be beneficial."

How do you know if you have parasites? A few of the symptoms are:

- Bluish color in the whites of your eyes
- Itching in the rectum area
- Fingernails that are brittle, hard and are concave, curving upward

Poor digestion

Food digestion is the responsibility of many organs in the body - the mouth, stomach, liver, gallbladder, spleen, pancreas, small intestine, and colon.

When food is not broken down where it can be absorbed through the small intestine, it will continue to your colon. There in your colon bad bacterium will break it down causing your colon to become more alkaline. This change in pH will reduce the good bacteria population, which will eventually lead to constipation.

Postponing a bowel movement

Each time you have an urge to have a bowel movement and don't head for the bathroom, you are training yourself to be constipated. This does not happen overnight but over many years of practice.

Delaying bowel movements can be a result of:

- Being in someone else's home
- Being where bathrooms are not readily available
- Not being able to use other's bathroom but your own
- Only going to the bathroom, when, everything is to your satisfaction.

So here's happens when you delay the urge to go to the bathroom. When your rectum is empty, it is collapsed. From the sigmoid colon, fecal matter enters the rectum; fills it, and you get a desire to have a bowel movement. If you ignore this desire too long, the nerves in the rectum wall lose their sensitive to the fecal matter irritation and pressure.

As the fecal matter sits in the rectum, more moisture is pulled out of the fecal matter by the rectum walls. The fecal matter becomes harder and harder the longer you delay your bowel movement. To remove this hard fecal matter, you will have to strain to push it out. Straining and puffing to have a bowel movement will cause rectal blood vessels to enlarge and cause excessive pressure on other organs.

Pregnancy

Being pregnant can cause you to be constipated. As the fetus grows, it starts to put pressure on the stomach, intestines, and rectum.

Use of prescription drugs

One side of effect of some calcium channel blocker is constipation – Calan, Isoptin. Drugs like Amitril, Elavil, Endep, Janimine, Surmontil, Tofranil and Vivactil that are used to treat depression can cause constipation.

Other drugs that can cause constipation are:

- Antacids

- Anticonvulsants
- Anticholinergics
- Antihypertensives
- Antidepressants
- Anti-parkinsonism
- Anti-psychotics
- Muscle relaxants
- Opiates
- Diuretics
- Iron salts

Feed the Good Bacteria

The good bacteria, in your colon, are known by many names – good bacteria, micro flora, and probiotics. This bacterium is necessary for good colon and body health. The main bacteria in your colon are:

- Lactobacillus acidophilus
- Bifidobacterium bifidum
- Lactobacillus salivarius
- Bifidobacterium infantis
- Streptococcus faecium

When buying probiotics buy a mixture of these bacteria. In some products you will find added **Fructo-oligosccharides**, **FOS**, which helps to feed the good bacteria and promote their survival.

Cultured yogurt is a good way to get additional good bacteria into your colon. The best way to eat it is in-between meals. The best yogurt to eat is goat milk yogurt. It costs a bit more but it is worth the health benefits you get from it. Look for yogurt that says the bacteria culture was added after pasteurization. If the yogurt was pasteurized after the bacteria culture was added, these good bacteria would have been destroyed.

Eat yogurt at least 3 times a week. You can add flax seed oil, berries, raisins, flax seed grounds, or other toping that promotes bowel movements.

The best way to get probiotics or good bacteria into your colon is to take a supplement, liquid or pill, between meals with distilled water. When probiotics are taken with food, food increases the stomach acid, which destroys the probiotic supplement.

Eating cultured vegetables is another way to get probiotics or good bacteria. Some flora-enhanced foods are:

- Sauerkraut
- Yogurt
- Kefir
- Miso
- Mico algae

Taking a Good Mineral Supplement

To maintain a strong and active colon, you need to take a good mineral supplement, which contain plenty of sodium, magnesium, calcium, and potassium. In addition, you need to get these minerals from the food you eat. Food has a balance of these minerals and nutrient you need to build your colon and other parts of your body.

Potassium

Potassium is needed to keep your colon walls working properly and for keeping them free of acid, which attracts disease. It helps to dislodge colon wastes that accumulate along your colon walls.

Potassium tastes bitter so most of the foods that are bitter contain potassium, especially herbal teas. Best foods to eat for high levels of potassium are:

Cucumbers	apples
Bitter greens	apple cider vinegar
Lentils	apricots
Almonds	bananas
Oatmeal	beans
Potato skins	blueberries
German prunes	goat milk
American prunes	grapes
Peaches	pears
Gooseberries	raisins
Romaine lettuce	tomatoes
Figs	sesame seeds
Carrots	beets and prunes

Prepare a Miracle Mineral Salad

Cut up romaine or dark green lettuce Chopped garlic cloves and onions 2-3 tablespoons of apple cider vinegar add hard-boiled eggs.

The allicin in the garlic is invigorated by the minerals in the onion and the allicin penetrates the large intestine wall. The fiber in the green vegetables helps to scrub the intestinal walls. The vinegar boosts enzymatic action of the allicin and the allicin stimulates the peristaltic movement. This is a natural way to dissolve accumulated toxic wastes on your colon wall and eliminate them.

To make this salad more potent make a salad dressing by combining.

- the juice to two cloves of garlic
- 2 tablespoon of flaxseed oil
- 3 tablespoons of olive oil
- 1 tablespoon of balsamic vinegar
- 2 tablespoons of apple cider vinegar
- ground up flax seeds, sunflower seeds
- one tablespoon of bran

Digestive enzymes

Digestive enzymes help you digest and absorb your food and supplements. Your body produces different enzymes to digest different types of food such as,

- Protease – for digesting protein
- Lactase – for digesting lactose a protein in milk
- Amylase – for digesting carbohydrate
- Pepsin – for digesting protein

- not use digestive enzymes if you have problems with ulcers.

Amylase starts carbohydrate digestion in your mouth. The longer you chew your food, which is a healthy practice, the better digested your food will be. Your stomach will not have to work as hard and less undigested food will reach your colon

Fruits and vegetables have their own digestive enzymes, which help to digest their selves. When fruits or vegetables are heated above 120 F, their enzymes are destroyed and no longer available for your body. When this happens, your body has to create these enzymes to digest this cooked food. This takes energy and enzymes away from within your body that could be used elsewhere to do more important work.

When you eat cooked food, processed and packaged foods, you use excessive digestive enzymes. Sometimes not all your food is digested properly and these undigested remains move into your colon where they create gas, toxic material, which weakens your colon wall.

Pregnant

If you are pregnant, here is a way to start your or assist your bowel movement. When sitting on the toilet, raise your legs to the same level of the toilet seat by placing your legs on a chair. Lean back slightly and place your arms above your head. You can also try to moving left and right to help the movement you need in the sigmoid and rectum to produce a bowel movement.

11: Powerful Ways to Stop & Overcome Constipation

Where to Start

I have given you plenty of information on how to relieve your constipation and how to prevent it. Just by applying many of the health ideas and tips that I have given, you are well on your way to creating excellent health and, of course, relieving your constipation.

I know that some of you will be confused about what to do first or where to start.

Each one of you will start by using different remedies. The ones you choose would depend on what you are familiar with, what you like to eat, what you have on hand, or how severe you are constipated.

A program to help you have regular bowel movements and to help you prevent having constipation consists of some basic steps.

From the information and remedies I have discussed in the previous chapters, you can experiment and test different ones and use the ones that work best for you.

In the case where you have had long-term constipation, it may be necessary to retrain your colon to have bowel movements. If this is the case, you may have to consult your doctor or an alternative medicine practitioner to get their direction

To get relief from frequent or occasionally constipation, these are the steps and changes you need to consider.

- Chose a natural laxative to relieve your constipation
- Eliminate constipating habits
- Improve your digestion
- Improve your diet
- Keep your good bacteria dominant in your colon
- Make your colon acidic
- Retrain your bowels for regularity
- Strengthen colon and surrounding areas

Choose a natural laxative to relieve you

constipation

Which natural laxative should you choose? I would recommend you choose 3 different ways to start relieving your constipation and use them at the same time.

First, I would recommend using Tripahal. Use it as directed on the bottle.

Second, start adding more fiber to your diet. If you eat oats or multigrain cream cereal, add bran to it. Or grind up some flax seed, sunflower seeds, sesame seeds or almonds and add it to your cereal.

Third, add a juice or vegetable remedy you like and use it every day for a week or so. Eat more fruits daily.

One of the methods that I use is taking 2 capsules of each cayenne pepper and MSM after each meal. I also drink apple juice, eat 2 apples each day, eat other fruits, eat oats, and various seeds. And of course, I eat fresh vegetables every day. There are other foods that I eat and those are listed in the chapters you have just read.

Eliminate Constipating Habits

Look at what constipating habits you have. Start changing them one by one. For example, on the first week you could concentrate on drinking more water. Start taking a quart of water to work in a glass jar. Add a small amount lemon to it to give a little flavor.

During the following week concentrate on eating more fruits and vegetables. Start taking apples to work or strips of carrots, celery, or other vegetables you like for snacks.

On the third week, you could concentrate on making and eating an evening salad every day of that week, if you are not already doing this.

On the fourth week, start adding more fiber to your diet.

Look at some of the other areas you need to change.

- Stop using Drugstore laxatives
- Start exercising more
- Drink more water
- Start going to the rest room when you have the urge for a bowel movement

These are the constipating habits you need to change. Start changing these habits one by one. Each day look at the list of habits to change and increase or decrease the habit as necessary.

Improve your digestion

By improving your digestion, you stop undigested food from reaching your colon where it can become putrefied.

You can help your digestion and improve your body's health by taking digestive enzymes at each meal. Taking digestive enzymes is almost a must for the elderly. They typically lack HCL acid to digest protein and need to take an HCL- pepsin supplement. And it would not hurt to take a regular enzyme supplement with it.

Improve your diet

There is no doubt you need to change your diet. If you have constipation, consider the main reason you do is eating the wrong kinds of food.

Fiber

Eating food with plenty of fiber is a requirement. There are many fruits and vegetables with plenty of fiber. You need to eat those foods that have plenty of soluble and non-soluble fiber. Eating only fruits and vegetable that contain mainly soluble fiber will not help you prevent or to stop constipation.

You also need those foods with plenty of non-soluble fiber, which adds bulk, draws water, and adds density to your stools. This type of fiber helps your fecal matter to move through your colon easier and quicker.

Bran

Bran is helpful in providing non-soluble fiber quickly to your eating program. Using the coarse fiber is better than the fine fiber. It is better to use plain bran rather than cereals with added bran. But in case you cannot find raw bran, then a second choice are cereals that contains processed bran and are high in fiber. Use this second choice bran only until your constipation is cleared.

It is better to use rice, oat, or corn bran rather than wheat bran. Mix the bran in your morning cereal – rolled oats, multigrain cereal

- pancakes, smoothies, salads, and wherever you feel it will taste good.

How much fiber should you eat? Eat between 30 – 40 mg of fiber every day. Fiber is one of the keys to keeping free of constipation.

If you are doing all the right things for improving the flow of fecal matter through you colon, and you still have constipation, then you need to see your doctor. This might be a sign of some underlying illness where you need a doctor's help.

Keep your good bacteria dominant in your colon. Keeping your good bacteria dominant in your colon can be difficult if you have become unbalance with excessive bad bacteria. The first step you need to take is to start feeding your good bacteria. You can do this by using edible dairy whey or FOS. You should also start eating those foods that feed the good bacteria.

In cases where you have used medical drugs for a long time, drink alcohol, use drugstore laxatives, or have been constipated for some time, you may have to resort to implanting good bacteria into your colon using an enema.

The technique for this has been discussed in Dave Webster's book, Acidophilus and Colon Health.

Make your colon acidic

Making and keeping your colon acidic requires you eat the right kind of food, have good digestion, and have a good mental attitude. The foods you should be eating are listed in the previous chapters. When you eat processed foods with little fiber and excess food additives, this changes your colon from acidic to an alkaline and helps the bad bacteria to multiple.

Keeping a negative attitude and having anxiety, also affects your colon. A continual tightening of your colon walls overworks your colon and eventually weakens it. A weaken colon is more susceptible to constipation which favors the growth of bad bacteria.

Retrain your bowels for regularity

Long-term constipation can come from your colon's inability to create peristaltic movement. This can result from long-term use of laxatives, use of pharmaceutical drugs, ignoring the signal to have a bowel movement, eating excessive process food, lack of fiber in your diet, and having excessive tension in your life.

To retrain your colon to have regular bowel movements, start by,

- Eating your meals at the same time every day
- Sit down on the toilet at the same time every morning and midday
- Use a herbal combination laxative that will gentle stimulate peristaltic action
- Consider learn some relaxation techniques to lessen any anxiety or tension you may be experiencing
- Follow the list of other actions to take to reduce constipation in this chapter.
- Use natural laxatives to help retrain and strengthen bowels

Strengthen colon and surrounding areas

How do you strengthen your colon? Getting the proper amount of minerals, vitamins, and oils into your body does this. Minerals help to build body cells and tissue. Use a mineral supplement like Alkalife or any other electrolyte type liquid mineral. Get your oils by using olive and flax oil in your salads and soups.

Exercise

No exercise is an unhealthy practice. Body movement in the abdominal area is necessary for good colon health. This movement comes from exercise such as running, walking, sit-ups, massage, and yoga stomach movements.

Exercise helps to tone and build colon wall tissue and muscle. It helps in moving fecal matter through your colon since exercise stretches and contracts your colon similar to what happens during peristaltic action.

The exercise I like is rebounding. This is one of the best exercises since it helps tone the whole body and activate your lymphatic system so your body fluid move easily.

Final Comments

As you change your diet, especially if you add more juices, fruits, and vegetables, you are going to experience cleansing of your body. What this means is you will experience some pain throughout your body as toxins are **released** and look for a way out of your body. As toxins come out of your cells and organs their acidity causes pain. Your body's minerals will neutralize some of this acid. That is why it is important to use a mineral supplement.

You may experience more mucus discharge as these toxins work their way out of your elimination ports. You may experience more mucus coming out of your nose, throat, and mouth. Mucus will also find its way into your colon and out the rectum in stools.

During this cleansing period, do not take any medication to stop or eliminate nasal drainage.

You may also develop rashes or other skin eruptions as toxins try to come out through your skin.

I leave you with the words of Fred S. Hirsch who wrote in 1975, in his small green booklet, "Constipation is a clogging-up of the entire human pipe-system. Nature wisely stores the undigested, toxic wastes "temporarily" in the tissues, awaiting an early opportunity to dispose of these poisons! Sickness is such an opportunity – "acute disease" is Nature's attempt to eliminate the stored-up "sewage" and the "healing process" differs according to the physical condition of each individual"

12: Additional Information on Constipation

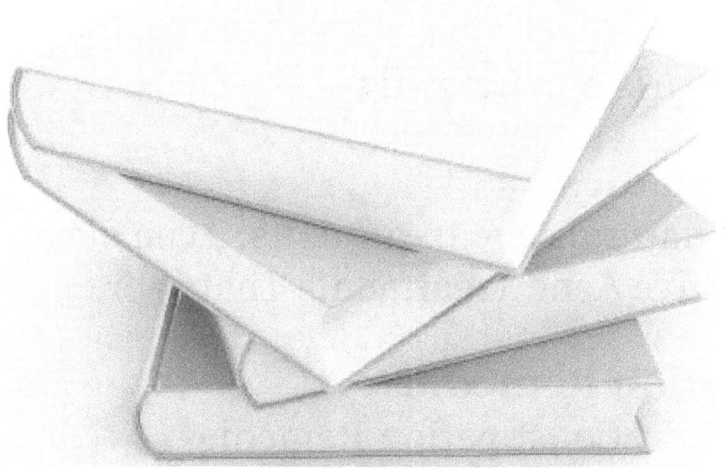

Get one of my best kindle books *free* below:

http://www.natural-remedies-thatwork.com

Christopher Teller is a natural nutritional consultant educated in the United States in Nutrition and Physics. He is a graduate from San Jose State University in California. He is author of 45 other books on natural remedies. He has authored a newsletter in natural remedies for over 10 years.

Resource page

Here are some of the other kindle e-books about natural remedies that have been written by this author. You can see the entire list at:

http://tinyurl.com/b2f7wd3

Acne Remedies
- Best natural acne treatments: Acne facial
- Effective Acne Treatments That Work

Constipation Remedies
- The Best Constipation Remedies
- Best Constipated Women Natural Cures
- How To Relieve Constipation With Fruits

Essential Fatty Acids
- Taking The Mystery Out Of Essential Fatty acids
- Amazing Fish Oil Benefits Revealed
- Omega 3 and 6 Mystery Exposed

Nutrition Remedies

- Updated Version - Secret Diet And Nutrition
- Secret Healthy Fruit Practices Revealed
- Fast Healing Juice Nutrition Therapy: Nutrition Tips 3
- Fantastic Alkaline Fruit Benefits Revealed
- Calcium (Discover How To Use Calcium To Avoid Devastating Diseases)
- Magnesium Nutrition Revealed
- Best Nutrition Health Practices
- Potassium Health Secrets Revealed
- Phosphorus, The Best Brain Food
- A Sodium Diet (What You Must Know About Sodium)
- Vegetables and Vegetable Juice Cures
- Alkaline Body: How to Change an Acid Body into an Alkaline body

Stomach Remedies

- Acid Reflux: Fast and Easy Cures For Acid Reflux
- Asthma Treatment Cures With Remedies
- How To Do Natural Colon Cleansing
- Gastrointestinal Digestion Secrets Revealed

Misc. Remedies

- Natural Hair Loss Treatment: Women And Men
- Effective Natural Hemorrhoids Treatment
- Iron Deficiency Anemia
- Secrets To Understanding Behavior
- Fast Acting Ear Infection Remedies
- Best Behavior Secrets Revealed That Can Change Your Personality
- What Is A Hiatus Hernia
- Best Varicose Vein Treatments?
- Make Shampoos At Home Using Natural Ingredients: Discover recipes for quality natural hair shampoos
- How To Fix Your Thyroid Problems: Discover Hidden Ideas That Fix Your Thyroid
- Nail Fungus & Health Treatment: Fix Your Fingernail's Health And Look Beautiful
- Gout Diet: New Ideas For Gout Treatments and Gout remedies for Eliminating Uric Acid and giving Gout Relief
- Diarrhea: How To Stop Diarrhea Chronic Or Severe

Minerals

- Calcium and Magnesium Magic Body Benefits Revealed
- The Magic of Sodium, Calcium and Magnesium
- Create an Alkaline Body with Potassium and Sodium: Eliminate a Potassium Deficiency
- Calcium and Phosphorus Foods: Deficiency or Excesses in These Minerals Cause Bone and Brain Power Loss

Men's Health
- Best Impotence Health Diet

Weight loss
- Ten (10) Day Quick Success Weight Loss Program: A new approach to losing weight by changing your eating habits for life
- Discover Secret Anti-Aging Juice & Tonic Recipes: Unique Juices And Tonics That Create Beauty And Youth

To see all of the kindle books written by this author, go to this the Authors Profile Page or this URL:
http://tinyurl.com/b2f7wd3

If you need support or want to promote any of his e-books, please contact him at rss41@yahoo.com and expect a reply within 24 hours. He looks forward to hearing from you and is happy to help you understand his material on natural and nutritional health.

Give A Review

And, don't for get to give a review for this e-book at Amazon so that others can gain the benefits of what is in this e-book. To you, for losing weight, creating better health and more happiness in your life,

Christopher Teller